PRAISE FOR THE CINEMATHERAPY SERIES

"Hilarious observations...A must for your next girls' night in."
—*Entertainment Weekly* (grade A-)

"This smart, sassy guide shows you how to overcome any mood by indulging in a film."—*Us*

"A cultural phenomenon."—*USA Today*

"It's like a session with a clever, movie-obsessed relationship therapist, with sharp insights into the psyche (at least as played out in films). And better yet, it rarely opts for the obvious choice to make the point, often favoring a more obscure, film-literate (and wiser) one."—*Premiere* magazine

"Fun, smart."—*Chicago Tribune*

"This tongue-in-cheek video guide rivals Siskel and Ebert in their prime."
—*Nebraska State Paper*

"A treasure and filled with wonderful surprises on every page. It's a 'must-have' for movie fans, but even if you don't watch movies, the book is fun to read."
—*Santa Monica Bay Week*

"Trade the therapist's couch for your own with the help of *Cinematherapy*."
—*Self*

"Brassy, sassy, and done with tongue planted firmly in cheek...Bona fide issues are addressed and real points made, but you know West and Peske are having fun."—*Denver Post*

"Hilarious."—*Pages*

"You could pay $100 an hour for real therapy—or you could go for the cheap 'n' easy alternative, compliments of Nancy Peske and Beverly West."—*Glamour*

"Clever...witty."—*Miami Herald*

"Offers not-always-obvious suggestions for, and pithy thumbnails of, great chick-flicks..."—*Fort Worth* [TX] *Morning Star Telegram*

"Fun."—*Body & Soul*

"A fun read and a great female-friendly guide for movie buffs." —*Weight Watchers* magazine

"Movies as medication."—*Toronto Sun*

"Peske and West know their movies."—*Daily Breeze*

"Lighthearted...breezy, chatty style."—*Publishers Weekly*

"A specialized version of Leonard Maltin, suggesting movies as a way to combat the blues."—*Hackensack* [NJ] *Record*

"Irreverent."—*Style Weekly*

"It's nicely done and, like a cup of fresh popcorn, really hard to put down." —*Hartford Courant*

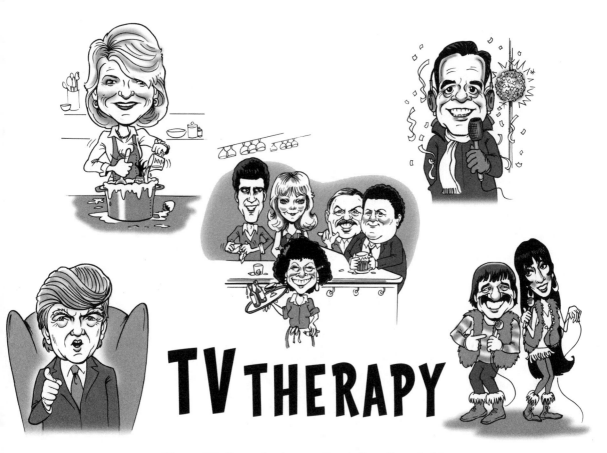

TV THERAPY

The Television Guide to Life

Beverly West and Jason Bergund

DELTA TRADE PAPERBACKS

TVTHERAPY
A Delta Trade Paperback / September 2005

Published by
Bantam Dell
A Division of Random House, Inc.
New York, New York

Delta is a registered trademark of Random House, Inc., and the colophon is a
trademark of Random House, Inc.

Library of Congress Cataloging-in-Publication Data
West, Beverly, 1961–
TVTherapy: the television guide to life/Beverly West and Jason Bergund
p. cm.
Includes index.
ISBN 0-385-33902-X
I. Television programs—United States—Catalogs. I. Bergund, Jason.
II. Title.

PN1992.3U5 W44 2005   2005045489

791.43/75/0973 22

Printed in the United States of America
Published simultaneously in Canada

www.bantamdell.com

RRH   10 9 8 7 6 5 4 3 2 1

To TV pioneers everywhere, who come into our family rooms every night to remind us that we're not alone

ACKNOWLEDGMENTS

Bev and Jason wish to thank Danielle Perez, the best editor and friend in the whole wide world, who has the added benefit of being the only person we know who knows more about TV than we do. Danielle, you are a rock star. We would also like to thank Preston Lindsay for his beautiful illustrations, which have added so much to our book. A very special thanks to our agent Jenny Bent for her creativity, support, and encouragement, not to mention her impeccable taste in heels; and to Michelle "Daisy Buchanan" Blakelely, who is always there to help us beat back the wolf from the door, and looks fabulous in fringe. You guys are all our shining stars.

Bev and Jason would also like to give a shout out to our extended TV family: Kristen Kreft, Geoffrey Barnes, Jessica Alonso, Ron Hayden, Kim Doi, Josh Kent, Amy Kent, Sadie Jones, Chris Lea, Arnie Mejia, Jen Star, Justin Hibner, Lauren Wong, Richard Ogawa, Kristopher Monroe, John Stanczyk, George Martino, Gretchen Krull, Brenda Cross, Aubyn Peterson, Tom Pennacchin, John Cameron Barnett, John Giuliano, Pam and Lily "You're Fired" Eisermann, Marilyn Adams, and Todd Jackson. Thanks to all of you for sharing so many wonderful moments just kicking back and watching the tube with us.

Jason:
Thanks to my family, especially my grandparents Pat and Stella Holden for letting me stay up late and watch our favorite TV shows, and for always being there with unconditional

love and support. Thanks also to my parents John and Darlene Bergund. A very special thank-you to my partner, Bev; you are the light of my life and I love you.

Bev:
Thanks to the all-seeing Joe Kolker, my parents Marilyn and Bill Knox, and to the newest addition to our personal TV generation, my nephew Jake. A special thanks to Ellen Rees and David Olds for their support, encouragement, and their generous contributions to the recently unveiled Ellen Rees Memorial Kitchen. And a very special thanks to my partner and TV guru Jason, who fills my life with love, laughter, and tons of great trash TV.

TABLE OF CONTENTS

INTRODUCTION

AT LAST! A home theater companion for all of us in the TV generation who understand that television is far more than just a pleasant diversion from the daily grind; it's a way of life. Our favorite shows are best friends and a form of remote-control therapy that can help us cope with everything from a bad-hair day to a bad breakup.

Television keeps us company when we're lonely, picks us up when we're blue, and encourages us to laugh at our troubles and unwind after a tough day at the office by watching some other poor schmuck hear the words "You're fired!"

Now, with the advent of DVD-TV, On Demand TV, TiVo, and satellite TV, for the first time in television history, do-it-ourselves televisiontherapists like us can pick and choose from the entire television pharmacy of home remedies and make our own decisions about what's on the tube tonight.

Suffering from a bad case of the dysfunctional family flu? Break bread with some of TV's favorite families, like the Sopranos, the Huxtables, or the Osbournes, and learn from the best, and the worst, how to make peace.

Experiencing a few growing pains? Embrace your inner adolescent with some Teen Spirit TV like *Jackass*, *South Park*, or *My So-Called Life*, and vent some of that pent-up angst without having to face a judge in the morning. Tired of winding up with the short end of the stick? Strike back with some TV justice like *CSI*, *Judge Judy*, or *L.A. Law*, and even the score.

TVTHERAPY: The Television Guide to Life also includes fun and informative sidebars like *Disastertherapy*, featuring some of reality television's most memorable messes; *Jason's Minibar,* with drink recipes to wet your whistle; *Bev's TV Tray*, offering incredible edibles guaranteed to feed your need; and timeless quotes from TV sages down through the ages, who can teach us all a thing or two about life on and off the air.

So whether you're on the verge of your nineteenth nervous breakdown, ready to exert some creative control, or searching for deeper meaning, *TVTHERAPY* will give you the guidance you need to find the right television prescription to match your mood, cure your malaise, or make your night, without ever getting up off the couch.

Send us your favorite TV prescriptions! You can e-mail the authors at: TVtherapy@ aol.com.

TVTHERAPY

CHAPTER 1

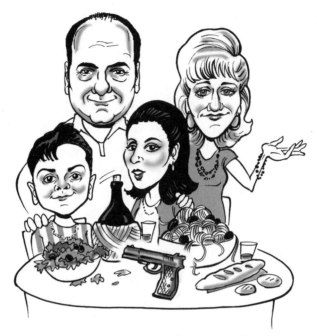

Dysfunctional Family TV

SURE YOU LOVE THEM, but there's just no denying that where there's family, there's bound to be fire every once in a while, and the warm embrace of home can begin to feel a lot like a nuclear event. Fortunately, at times like these we can always turn to the greatest family fire retardant ever invented, family TV, to help us turn down the heat, or at least distract us long enough to forget what we were bickering about. So when your nuclear family reactor is approaching critical mass, cool off together in front of the tube with some Dysfunctional Family TV, featuring TV families that reflect the best and the worst in all of us, and remember that the family that watches TV together stays together, at least for thirty minutes minus commercial breaks.

■ *The Sopranos* (1999–)
   Stars: *James Gandolfini, Edie Falco, Lorraine Bracco, Michael Imperioli,*
      Robert Iler, Jamie-Lynn DiScala

If there's trouble brewing in your family compound and you're ready to go to the mattresses, let *The Sopranos* reassure you that no matter how much excess baggage your dysfunctional family members are lugging around, at least they aren't packing heat.

The Sopranos picks up where *The Godfather* left off, and offers us all a front-row recliner in the life of a suburban Mafia family that has one foot in a Sam's Club brand of social acceptability, and the other planted waist deep in the vendetta-soaked soil of the Italian underworld. And what we discover is that where dysfunctional families are concerned, no matter which direction you go, you invariably wind up in Sicily.

Carmela (Edie Falco) and Tony Soprano (James Gandolfini) are suburban soccer parents who worry about their kids, their retirement, and what the neighbors think. Carmela is a good Catholic who bakes the best ziti in the neighborhood, wonders if this is all there is, still looks damn good in a pair of capris and a double-knit twin set, and overdoses daily on denial. And Tony…well…Tony is definitely pushing the outside limits of his shirt seams, in more ways than one. Thrown into the mix are two overindulged teens, a *famiglia*-size anxiety disorder, a mother-in-law engaged in a lifelong performance of *St. Joan of the Stockyards*, an overly involved psychiatrist, and a flaky sister who is perpetually losing herself in alternative religions and really, really bad relationships.

In short, the only difference between the Sopranos and the average American family is that when this tribe experiences feelings of homicidal rage, it's not just a fantasy, and the elephants in the Soprano family room are usually carrying automatic weapons.

What makes *The Sopranos* such strong medicine for all of us with a bad case of the dysfunctional *famiglia* flu is the reassurance that while this family has grappled with just about every serious family nightmare you can think of, they have nevertheless managed to stay together and alive for five seasons and counting.

Once you get past the vendettas, the extortion rackets, the pinkie rings, the Bada-Bing girls, and the extremely bad suits, you find a family that is learning, in a new way each week, that what you don't know really can hurt you, and that the ancient code of silence or death is not really such a good idea where family dynamics are concerned. The Sopranos' struggle for survival teaches us all that fighting is not always such a bad thing, because the family that stays together is the family that can talk openly and honestly with each other, safe in the knowledge that they will never be whacked by the people that they trust most. So if your family has put out a contract on you, show up with a big pan of ziti and share a season of *The Sopranos*, then break some bread, talk things through, and make the peace Sicilian style.

SOPRANO FAMILY JEWELS

Look, this thing of ours, the way it's going, it'd be better if we could admit to each other these painful, stressful times. But it'll never fucking happen.
★ Steve Van Zandt as Silvio Dante in *The Sopranos*

There's an old Italian saying: you fuck up once, you lose two teeth.
★ James Gandolfini as Tony Soprano in *The Sopranos*

What, no fucking ziti?
★ Robert Iler as A. J. Soprano in *The Sopranos*

DISASTERTHERAPY

Growing Up Gotti (2004)
Stars: Victoria Gotti, Frank Agnello, John Agnello, Carmine Agnello Jr.

If you're feeling overwhelmed by your mob, pay a visit to Victoria Gotti's house, where every day is a struggle for control, and be reassured that as hot as things get in your family pressure cooker, they could definitely get hottier. Victoria, daughter of the late Teflon don John Gotti, is a single working mom trying to pull in the reins on her three rambunctious teenage boys. And while Victoria and her famiglia live in a traditional manse by the sea that is straight out of an Ethan Allen wet dream, the lunatics are definitely in charge of the family room. In hottie Gotti land, hair gel is a cause for full-out war, English sounds like a foreign language, and etiquette is a village in France that nobody visits anymore. Ironically, as this is a show about growing up after all, the most unruly teenager in the brood is Victoria herself, who for all of her Gotti bluster and bravado doesn't have the moxie to carry through on any of her threats. And so it falls to her boys to govern themselves in a world where words speak far louder than action. It's no wonder that everybody shouts.

VICTORIA'S VENDETTAS

I'm gonna cook. Bring the Kaopectate.

I am neurotic and you will put me in a mood like you cannot imagine.

If you were my daughter I would take you by your hair, and I would swing you around a coupla times.

Everybody better pay attention because I am not kidding. Whoever breaks this rule will be put on a plane back home and I will personally drive them to the airport.

Let me tell you something. If you're going on a job interview, at least take your piercings out.

★ all quotes from Victoria Gotti in *Growing Up Gotti*

- *The Addams Family* (1964–1966)
  Stars: *John Astin, Carolyn Jones, Ted Cassidy, Jackie Coogan, Marie Blake, Ken Weatherwax, Lisa Loring*
  Based on the New Yorker *cartoons by Charles Addams*

The Addams family—who live on Cemetery Lane, keep spiders for house pets, and cultivate carnivorous plants rather than roses—reassures us all that when it comes to family dynamics, even strange and exotic creatures of the night aren't all that different from the rest of us.

Morticia Addams (Carolyn Jones) is the wife and mom we all wish we had, and most women wish they could become. Morticia nurtures her children without smothering them, keeps the romance alive in her marriage, and still fits into her wedding gown. She spends her days knitting for her cousins, feeding her plants, and fretting over her design motif. That is, when Morticia isn't doing the tango with her dashing husband with a bullwhip in her hand.

And dad, Gomez Addams (John Astin), is a rich and rakish lawyer who lives in his smoking jacket and never has to leave his living room. He spends lots of quality time with his kids, is still passionately in love with his wife, and uses his brother-in-law for target practice whenever he isn't dancing a passionate merengue with his wife with a rose clutched in his teeth. Now, that's our kind of gender bending.

But what we love best about the Addamses is that they don't seem to give a second thought to what anybody else thinks of them. Like true Victorians, they feel completely entitled to be as grotesque and flagrantly freakish on the outside as we all secretly feel on the inside . . . and don't see anything odd about themselves at all. The Addamses don't hide their eccentricities, they indulge them, and teach us that the best family home is the one where all members feel appreciated and accepted for who and what they are, even if they're a thing or an it. *The Addams Family* reminds all our family ghosts that no matter how creepy or kooky, mysterious or ookie, we're all still family, no matter what the neighbors think.

ADDAMS FAMILY JEWELS

I'm quite proud of Mrs. Addams's hothouse. She's raised these plants from tiny weeds.
★ John Astin as Gomez Addams in *The Addams Family*

Somebody down there likes me!
★ John Astin as Gomez Addams in *The Addams Family*

I've been yours since that first day you carved my initials in your leg.
★ Carolyn Jones as Morticia Addams in *The Addams Family*

■ *The Munsters* (1964–1966)
Stars: Fred Gwynne, Yvonne De Carlo, Al Lewis, Beverley Owen,
Pat Priest, Butch Patrick

If you're in the midst of a family horror show, spend a few hours with the Munsters, a family of Frankensteins, werewolves, and vampires, which nevertheless manages to be one of the most functional families on the teleblock.

The Munsters, which was created by the same folks who brought us *Leave It to Beaver*, turns the suburban family ideal on its ear and gives us a family of monsters who know a lot more about family dynamics than their "normal" counterparts. Unfortunately, the neighbors can't see past the Munsters' undead appearance to their living hearts of gold. And unlike their creepy sitcom family rivals, the Addamses, who could care less what the neighbors think, the Munsters try to keep up with the Joneses. Episode after episode finds the Munsters struggling for social acceptance and succeeding only in winning over each other, and reminding us all in the process that it's who a family is on the inside, and not what they look like on the outside, that matters in the end.

MUNSTER FAMILY JEWELS

Herman tried to build a ship inside a bottle. We had to break the bottle to get him out.

★ Yvonne De Carlo as Lily Munster in *The Munsters*

You better start dawdling to school, Eddie, or otherwise you will be on time.

★ Yvonne De Carlo as Lily Munster in *The Munsters*

■ *Diff'rent Strokes* (1978–1986)
  Stars: *Conrad Bain, Gary Coleman, Todd Bridges, Dana Plato,*
  Charlotte Rae

If you're like a mismatched ensemble in a twin-set world, let this family of coordinated separates remind you that it's not the color of the cloth but the tapestry of the heart that knits a family together.

When rich white guy Philip Drummond's (Conrad Bain) widowed African American maid passes away, her last request is that Mr. Drummond take care of the two young sons she is leaving behind her. And because this is TV-land in the late seventies, when Norman Lear had made anything possible, Arnold (Gary Coleman) and Willis (Todd Bridges) leave the hood and move in with Mr. Drummond, his teenage daughter, Kimberly (Dana Plato), and his new housekeeper, Mrs. Garrett (Charlotte Rae), and become a family. What ensues are plenty of antic life lessons about what it means to be a family. It all boils down to the heartfelt and hopeful message that people who are different colors, and from different backgrounds, can still be a family as long as they have love in common.

▪ *Sanford and Son (1972–1977)*
  Stars: Redd Foxx, Demond Wilson

If you're still stinging from your last smack-down with your perpetually disapproving patriarch, and you want to remember that underneath all that brass beats a heart of pure gold, go treasure hunting at the Sanford and Son Salvage Yard and let Fred Sanford (Redd Foxx) and his son, Lamont (Demond Wilson), remind you that all that rusts and creaks is not necessarily junk.

TV FAMILIES WE WISH WOULD ADOPT US

When you're wondering if you were adopted, or just wish you were, spend a couple of hours with one of our favorite functional TV families, because the best thing about being in charge of your own remote control is that you can choose your family.

Roseanne (1988–1997)
Stars: Roseanne Barr, John Goodman, Laurie Metcalf, Sara Gilbert, Lecy Goranson, Michael Fishman, Sarah Chalke

We'd like to grow up again with Roseanne's TV family, because through the Conners' eyes, dysfunctional family life seemed a little less diabolical and a lot, well, funnier. As the Conners work through the average life cycle of the new American family, they fall back on their heartland values of truth, tolerance, and a handful of really good one-liners, and somehow they make it through. The Conners give us permission to stop beating up on ourselves and take a load off. They reassure us that it's okay that we sometimes eat Twinkies for dinner, that money is often tight, that our window treatment does not coordinate fetchingly with our Barcalounger, and that while we may sometimes fall short of the American family ideal, at least we have each other.

CONNER FAMILY JEWELS

Oh, isn't that sweet? My son just closed his first drug deal.

Your idea of romance is popping the can away from my face.

Oh, look, honey, our kids are necking.

Marriage stinks with a capital SUCK.

Hold the knife steady, Dan, I keep missing my wrist.

★ all quotes from Roseanne Barr as Roseanne Conner in *Roseanne*

The Cosby Show *(1984–1993)*
*Stars: Bill Cosby, Phylicia Rashad, Lisa Bonet, Sabrina Le
Beauf, Malcolm-Jamal Warner, Tempestt Bledsoe,
Keshia Knight Pulliam*

Dr. Cliff Huxtable (Bill Cosby) is a successful OB/GYN who lives in a
restored brownstone with period detailing, in a great Brooklyn neighborhood in
New York City, along with his beautiful and brilliant wife Clair (Phylicia
Rashad), a lawyer, and his five incredibly well-scrubbed and well-mannered kids,
who are all on their way to Ivy League colleges. And if this sounds like a nuclear
family heaven on earth, you're right. The Huxtables are the most functional
family on the TV block. Nothing ever happens in the Cosby household that can't
be cured with a nod, a wink, or a Jell-O pudding pop, and a few words of kindly
but firm advice from Father Huxtable. Some have criticized *The Cosby Show* for
glossing over so many of the domestic and social issues that might have been
addressed in this sitcom about an African American family living the American
dream. But we think it's revolutionary by presenting a functional family that
transcends race, color, and creed in a show that managed to stay at the top of its
game for nearly a decade without having to resort to a rotating assortment of
guest stars or adopting a new child to keep the ratings up.

CLIFF'S NOTES

No boy should have a ninety-five-dollar shirt unless he is onstage with his four brothers!

You know, America is a great place, but it doesn't have a place where you can get rid of your kids.

I am sure, somewhere, there is a suit that goes with this tie. Don't get me the suit!

Let me tell you something. Your mother and I go into the kitchen. You can go out and get in my car. You can drive backwards to Coney Island, run over the hot dog man and two stop signs, and you won't be in any more trouble than you are in now.

This is Dr. Huxtable. I delivered some of you. I'm a parent and a taxpayer. And I am probably the only adult who will sue little children.
★   all quotes from Bill Cosby as Cliff Huxtable in *The Cosby Show*

The Osbournes (2002–2004)
Stars: Ozzy, Sharon, Kelly, and Jack Osbourne

First of all, we love the house! Second of all, just how many refillable prescriptions for euphorics are there just lying around that fabulous manse? And third, life in the Osbourne family has already gone to the dogs, so it takes a lot of the pressure off everybody right from the get-go. America's new-millennium Brady Bunch, whose lives are a lot like *The Rocky Horror Picture Show* meets *Martha Stewart Living*, is a great reminder that as weird as things can get on the surface, even a guy who used to bite the heads off bats onstage is really just a harmless Mike Brady underneath, only with an edgier stylist who has finally come out of the closet. The Osbournes reassure us that underneath the fright wigs that we all occasionally don to scare everybody away is the familiar face of home.

OZZY'S ODDBALLS

I'm not proud of everything I've done. I'm not proud of having a poor education. I'm not proud of being dyslexic. I'm not proud of being an alcoholic drug addict. I'm not proud of biting the head off a bat. I'm not proud of having attention deficit disorder. But I'm a real guy. To be Ozzy Osbourne. It could be worse, I could be Sting.

★ Ozzy Osbourne in *The Osbournes*

■ *Mama's Family (1983–1990)*
Stars: Vicki Lawrence, Ken Berry, Dorothy Lyman, Rue McClanahan,
Carol Burnett, Betty White, Beverly Archer

If your apple has rolled a long way from the family tree, and you're feeling homesick for some cheap wine and relatives, spend a few hours with *Mama's Family*, and remember that familiarity breeds not only contempt, but also perennial adolescence, narcissism, co-dependence, and often a pretty severe case of indigestion. And try though you may to sever the roots, the bonds of Mama's love are hard to loose.

Widow woman Thelma "Mama" Harper (Vicki Lawrence) is the matriarch of her extended rural Southern family (read white trash) who rules her roost with an iron tongue and solves every problem with a can of Bud, a slab of meat loaf, a smack upside the head, and a healthy dose of the unvarnished truth. And somehow, everything comes out all right in the end.

When Mama's middle-aged son Vinton (Ken Berry) moves back into her house with two kids, his main squeeze—emphasis on the word *squeeze*—Naomi (Dorothy Lyman), and enough family baggage to fill a double-wide, let's just say the glassware, and the small-town life lessons, really start to fly.

On the sidelines of this hometown smack-down are a carnival of visiting guest artists (who can all trace their roots back to *The Carol Burnett Show* family, where *Mama's Family* was created). There's Eunice (Carol Burnett), Mama's daughter on the verge of a nervous break-down, and Mama's spinster sister Aunt Fran (Rue McClanahan), who eventually dies while choking on a chicken bone, and her other daughter Ellen (Betty White), who "married up" and looks down on her humble origins.

But the strongest link in this dysfunctional family chain is Thelma herself, who vents her universal disapproval of just about anybody who's even distantly related to her, in a futile effort to preserve some dignified Dixie-style order amid the white-trash chaos that constantly threatens to engulf them all.

Mama's Family is a great antidote for the hometown blues, because it reminds us that while the family ties that bind might occasionally pinch, in the end they will also keep us from hitting the ground when we fall and breaking something really important. So when you need to remember where you came from, let *Mama's Family* reassure you that be it ever so trashy, there's no place like home.

MAMA KNOWS BEST

From now on if we have any backstabbing to do we're going to do it the way we have always done it, face-to-face.

The only way to keep from goin' crazy in this house is to stay half lit.

I tell ya, a guy selling brains could clean up in this family.

From now on, I'm not gonna give my family anything but hell!
★   all quotes from Vicki Lawrence as Mama in *Mama's Family*

■ *All in the Family (1971–1979)*
  Stars: Carroll O'Connor, Jean Stapleton, Sally Struthers, Rob Reiner

If the times they are a-changin' in your family pond, and you're feeling nostalgic for a simpler time when girls were girls and men were men, spend a few hours with the Bunker family, which will help you debunk the mythology of the good old days that never were.

Archie Bunker (Carroll O'Connor) is a middle-aged, borough-bred, and bigoted good old boy who is completely convinced of the righteousness of his position, and utterly misinformed. And more than anything else in the world, Archie hates change. In short, Archie is 1950s America made flesh. Archie lives with his doting but dotty wife, Edith (Jean Stapleton), his daughter, Gloria (Sally Struthers), who is the apple of his eye, and his son-in-law, Mike (Rob Reiner), who is the 1960s made flesh, and just about as annoying as a sit-in at rush hour.

Obviously, much antic family room combat ensues as Mike—who believes in peace, love, and understanding—and Archie—who believes in Barcaloungers, Richard Nixon, belching, and beer—battle it out on the front lines of the war between the old and the new version of the American family. And remarkably, despite the near-constant shouting, a generation gap the size of the Grand Canyon, the small-mindedness, and the excess intestinal gas, the Bunkers find a way to live together without killing each other and reach toward a more harmonious future for them all.

So when your home waters are rapidly rising, let *All in the Family* reassure you that as long as you love each other you can always find a way to start swimming before you sink like a stone.

ARCHIE'S APHORISMS

*That ain't the American way, buddy. With Lady Liberty standin'
there in the harbor, with her torch on high sayin' "Send me your poor,
your deadbeats, your filthy." And they all come spillin' in here, they
come swarming in like ants . . . your Spanish PRs . . . your Japs, your
Chinamen, your Krauts and your Hebes and your English fruits. They
all come spillin' in here where they're all free to live in their own sepa-
rate sections where they feel safe. And they'll bust your head if you go
in there. That's what makes America beautiful, buddy.*

I know all about your woman's troubles there, Edith, but when I had the hernia that time, I didn't make you wear the truss. If you're gonna have the change of life, you gotta do it right now. I'm gonna give you just thirty seconds. Now c'mon and change!

Whatever happened to the good old days when kids was scared to death of their parents?

★   all quotes from Carroll O'Connor as Archie Bunker in *All in the Family*

■ *The Jeffersons (1975–1985)*
Stars: Sherman Hemsley, Isabel Sanford, Roxie Roker, Franklin Cover, Marla Gibbs

If you're in the mood for a second scoop of family dysfunction New York style, move on up to the East Side to the Jeffersons' *dee*-luxe apartment in the sky. George Jefferson (Sherman Hemsley), who was Archie Bunker's next-door neighbor, hits it big with his chain of dry-cleaning stores and moves his family out of Queens and into a penthouse on the right side of the tracks. And in Manhattan that was saying a lot. Together with his lovable rock of a wife, Weezy (Isabel Sanford), his sarcastic son, Lionel (Mike Evans), and his sharp-tongued maid, Florence (Marla Gibbs), George tries to find a comfortable niche for himself and his family amid the upper crust of Madison Avenue. In the process, George and his family discover a new vision of the African American family, one that gets its turn at bat and winds up in the big leagues.

Bev's TV Tray:
Healthy Boundary Burritos

Has your emotional homeland been vulnerable to hostile invaders lately? Are your precious natural resources being siphoned off without anybody paying a tariff? Declare a trade embargo with this burrito, whose preparation is a great lesson in how to maintain clean boundaries so that your oil and water don't mix.

Here's what you'll need:

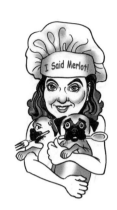

1 package Pillsbury crescent rolls

1 can refried beans (8 oz.)

1 cup cream cheese, softened

$\frac{1}{2}$ cup sour cream plus extra for garnish

2 tablespoons chile powder

1 teaspoon salt

1 cup grated cheddar cheese

2 cups canola oil for frying

Salsa

Sliced tomatoes, lettuce, and black olives

Fresh lime

Here's how you do it:

Roll out the crescent rolls until they are $\frac{1}{8}$ inch thick. Combine beans, cream cheese, sour cream, chile powder, and salt in a medium bowl and whip until light. Fill each crescent with the bean and cheese mixture, sprinkle with cheddar, then roll up, making sure to seal the burritos so that all of your borders are tight. Heat the oil in a medium skillet and fry the burritos on all sides until golden brown. This doesn't take long, maybe 3 or 4 minutes tops, so watch the pan closely. Top your burritos with a little salsa, some lime, a dollop of sour cream, and the tomatoes, lettuce, and black olives. Then bite into your burrito and let it all hang out.

FOOD FOR THOUGHT

After a good meal one can forgive anyone ... even one's relatives.

★ Oscar Wilde

▪ *The Simpsons (1989–)*
   Stars: Dan Castellaneta, Julie Kavner, Yeardley Smith,
      Nancy Cartwright, Hank Azaria, Harry Shearer

The Simpsons debuted in 1989 as America's first animated dysfunctional family, and has been putting the fun in dysfunction ever since. Homer (Dan Castellaneta) is an overweight, undereducated dad who works for a nuclear power plant and lives for his time off with his family and his Duff beer. Marge (Julie Kavner) is the power mom of the household, with a blue bouffant that could knock over buildings in a strong wind, and a Pall Mall voice that reminds us with every smoky syllable that the hand that stirs the pot can also light a match in a gale-force wind if necessary. And then of course there's Bart (Nancy Cartwright), everybody's favorite underachiever and the self-proclaimed Dennis the Menace for a new generation, who spends his life tormenting his father and trying to get something for nothing, and usually winding up getting what he's paid for.

Perhaps *The Simpsons* is the longest-running sitcom in TV history and still going strong because the politically and psychologically incorrect symptoms reassure us that we're all a mess once you scratch the surface, but as long as we love each other and do no real harm, we can forgive ourselves for falling a little short of the American family ideal.

HOMER'S HOMILIES

Weaseling out of things is important to learn. It's what separates us from the animals . . . except the weasel.

Maybe, just once, someone will call me "sir" without adding, "you're making a scene."

Kids, just because I don't care doesn't mean I'm not listening.

Son, when you participate in sporting events, it's not whether you win or lose: it's how drunk you get.

Lisa, if you don't like your job you don't strike, you just go in every day and do it really half-assed—that's the American way.

Kids, you tried your best and you failed miserably. The lesson is, never try.

It's not easy to juggle a pregnant wife and a troubled child, but somehow I managed to fit in eight hours of TV a day.

Alcohol, the cause of and the solution to all of life's problems.

★ all quotes from Homer Simpson in *The Simpsons*

WHAT'S WRONG WITH THIS PICTURE? PERFECT TV FAMILIES THAT WEREN'T REALLY SO PERFECT

Leave It to Beaver (1957–1963)
Stars: Hugh Beaumont, Barbara Billingsley, Tony Dow, Jerry Mathers

The Cleavers still hold on to top billing in the picture-perfect TV family hall of fame, and for good reason. Who wouldn't have wanted to grow up with a mom (Barbara Billingsley) who could vacuum and bake without creasing her crinoline and a dad (Hugh Beaumont) made entirely out of tweed, pipe tobacco, and good old-fashioned common sense, and dwell in a world where the biggest problems are what to do with found money and whether or not Beaver is ready to graduate out of his short pants. When you consider, though, that the Cleavers broadcast into a world where Martin Luther King Jr. was leading the Montgomery bus boycott, Castro seized power, Allen Ginsberg was penning *Howl*, Woody Guthrie was singing "This Land Is Your Land," Tennessee Williams won the Pulitzer for *A Streetcar Named Desire*, and Britain started developing atomic weapons, you have to kind of wonder just how great a job the Cleavers really did in preparing Wally (Tony Dow) and the Beav (Jerry Mathers) to become productive citizens of the world.

The Brady Bunch (1969–1974)
*Stars: Florence Henderson, Robert Reed, Ann B. Davis, Maureen McCormick,
Eve Plumb, Susan Olsen, Barry Williams, Christopher Knight, Mike
Lookinland*

The Bradys were the Cleavers for the next generation of kids who were
growing up in a world where families were not always born, but made … and
then remade. *The Brady Bunch*, just in case there's anyone who's been dwelling in
a cave for the last five decades and *doesn't* know the theme song, is based on the
story of a lovely lady, who was bringing up three very lovely girls. Then one day,
she meets a fella with three boys of his own, and they knew that it was much
more than a hunch that this group must somehow form a family, and this is
how we all became forever after transfixed by the utopia of denial that was *The
Brady Bunch*.

The Bradys managed to make blending a family look about as difficult as
folding bread crumbs into one of Alice's famous meat loaves, yet what came out
of the oven at the end didn't taste any different from what was cooking at the
Cleavers'. This comforted us in the short run, knowing that no matter what
kind of ingredients go into the bowl, it's all going to come out meat loaf in the
end. But we wonder what might have happened if the Bradys had embraced a
little of the summer of love/winter of our discontent world that lay beyond
their backyard fence. What if Carol had joined a consciousness-raising group?
Or if Greg had been drafted? Or what if, instead of developing a crush on Davey
Jones, Marsha had developed a thang for the Velvet Underground? Perhaps they
would have produced a new generation of gourmets who embraced a new kind
of melting pot, rather than insisting on the same old ground chuck.

The Partridge Family (1970–1974)
*Stars: Shirley Jones, David Cassidy, Susan Dey, Danny Bonaduce, Brian
Forster, Jeremy Gelbwaks, Suzanne Crough, Dave Madden*

Well, we know that it was really cool at the time to broadcast a show about a
single-parent family that dressed in Paul Revere and the Raiders hand-me-
downs and rode around on a bus together encouraging us all to come on and get

happy. But we wonder how healthy it was for Shirley to encourage her children to take the show on the road when the majority of her brood had no musical talent whatsoever. And what was with those ruffles on their shirts?

Full House *(1987–1995)*
Stars: Bob Saget, John Stamos, Dave Coulier, Mary-Kate Olsen, Ashley Olsen

Okay, we understand that a dad raising his kids alone was a socially responsible view of a new kind of American family. And Mary-Kate and Ashley are way cute; there's just no way around that. But we really do wonder about the constantly rotating assortment of big-haired babes placed in the living room to dilute the obviously homoerotic implication of three eighties-style disco dudes who harmonize best with one another, raising three little princesses in a world that is otherwise completely devoid of women.

Jason's Minibar—The '57 Chevy with Hawaiian Plates

The next time you're getting queasy on your dysfunctional family road trip, pull over at a rest stop, designate a different driver, indulge in this favorite family vacation elixir, and enjoy the view.

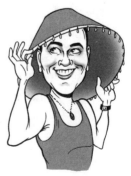

Here's what you'll need:
> *2 ounces Southern Comfort*
> *2 ounces vodka*
> *2 ounces orange juice*
> *2 ounces pineapple juice*
> *Dash grenadine*

Here's how you do it:
Shake all ingredients with ice in a cocktail shaker. Strain into a rocks glass with a couple of big ice cubes.

DISASTERTHERAPY

Showbiz Moms and Dads (2004)

From Fenton Bailey and Randy Barbato, the filmmakers who brought us *The Eyes of Tammy Faye* and the shockumentary *Party Monster*, comes a reality show that focuses an unrelenting lens on stage parents, who will stop at nothing to make their "children's" dreams of stardom come true, and remind us all in the process that it's better to languish in obscurity than to star in your parents' epic fantasies.

Showbiz Moms and Dads focuses on five stage families, headed up by controlling moms and deluded dads, who will stop at nothing, including fracturing their kids' superegos, in order to taste their fifteen minutes of fame. And let us tell you, this show is straight out of your own most horrific Warhol fantasies and makes for some good trash TV.

Debbie Klingensmith rehearses her thirteen-year-old son, Shane, in the basement to become the next teen sensation, without ever realizing that her pubescent son is starting to sound less like Justin Timberlake and more like Peter Brady in the Brady kids' rendition of "It's Time to Change." Debbie Tye troops her four-year-old JonBenet-Ramsey-double daughter, Emily, through a succession of teeny-weeny beauty pageants in the hopes of securing a teeny-weeny crown that will be much too small to fit on Mom's swelled head anyway. Tiffany Barron struggles with her own inner teenage celebrity when her fourteen-year-old daughter, Jordan, decides she is now ready for a close-up that doesn't include her mom. And then there are the Nutters, whose name just about says it all. The Nutters, seven kids and a seen but not heard mom, are guided by their egomaniacal father to leave Vermont in pursuit of his disappointed Barbra Streisand dreams and wind up in a small walk-up in Queens.

While this admittedly sounds like a great setup for a hit sitcom, we suspect that it will turn out too dark for prime time in the end. *Showbiz Moms and Dads* is a riveting look into the world of families that are in the process of selling their souls for fifteen minutes of fame, and reminds us all that it does not benefit us to gain the world if we lose our families.

The Surreal Life *(2003–)*

It's hard to argue with a reality show that creates an artificial family out of washed-up stars, puts them in a house that looks like it was designed by Hieronymus Bosch after a few drinks with Andy Warhol, and expects them to work out their family issues with each other. This surreal family psychodrama, featuring a rotating cast of marginal and generally psychologically oblivious and emotionally damaged celebrities (which have included Tammy Faye, Vanilla Ice, Brigitte Nielsen, Flavor Flav, Charo, Ron Jeremy, M. C. Hammer, and Emmanuel Lewis) is a great lesson in the unstoppable power of the family structure. No matter who is in the surreal house, the group always somehow forms a family. There is inevitably a father figure who emerges and tries to create a framework to keep his family safe, and who offers a cool head in times of crisis. And there's a mom figure, who offers unconditional wisdom and love, and a pack of unruly and spoiled children who will do whatever they can to ensure that they get the lion's share of Mom and Dad's attention. As these artificial families of sputtering stars scramble to muster a last twinkle in the twilight, we discover along with them that what we are longing for is the love and support of people who will love us for who we are underneath the surface sparkle, and that fame is a poor substitute for family.

CHARO'S CUCHI-CUCHIS

The first impression I get when I walk into this house is Liberace with diarrhea, 1940.

People alive don't understand me. How in the world a ghost is going to understand me?

I'm psychic. So I know whatever he's telling, he's full of shit.

I'm walking around and I see Brigitte Nielsen with her big tits hanging around. Oh, my God. I hope she doesn't think this is a surreal porno.

★ all quotes from Charo in *The Surreal Life*

HOME, HOME ON THE RANGE

If you're hungry for some old-fashioned family values, step back in time with these functional families of yesteryear that couldn't afford the luxury of family dysfunction. Because when you're sawing wood for a living way out where the deer and the antelope play, and your closest neighbor is two territories away, you have no choice but to get along with your relatives.

The Waltons *(1972–1981)*
Stars: Richard Thomas, Ralph Waite, Michael Learned, Ellen Corby, Will Geer, Judy Norton-Taylor, Jon Walmsley, Mary Beth McDonough, Eric Scott, David W. Harper, Kami Cotler, Mary Jackson, Helen Kleeb

The coming-of-age reminiscences of John Boy Walton (Richard Thomas), a young writer growing up in the bosom of an extended family in the Blue Ridge Mountains, captivated audiences in the seventies who were still stinging from the moral confusion of the summer of love and were longing to get back to the garden, and remind us all that one man's white trash is a network's treasure. On Walton's Mountain, where the only thing that's in abundance is relatives, this idealized TV family weathers the storms of poverty, youthful ambition, anti-Semitism, adult illiteracy, puppy love, and the temptations of Miss Mamie's evil recipe, and always manages to emerge the morning after with their roots still firmly planted in the Appalachian soil. What was it that made the Walton family so functional and so resilient that they beat out *The Mod Squad* and Flip Wilson to command their time slot? Perhaps it was John Walton's (Ralph Waite) velvet-voiced wisdom, Olivia's (Michael Learned) will of iron, or Grandma (Ellen Korby) and Grandpa's (Will Geer) curmudgeonly advice. Or maybe it was just really, really great acting.

Little House on the Prairie (1974–1983)
Stars: Michael Landon, Karen Grassle, Melissa Gilbert, Melissa Sue Anderson, Lindsay Sidney Greenbush

Charles Ingalls and his daughter, Half-pint (Melissa Gilbert), captivated television audiences for over a decade with the Michael Landon signature brand of homespun family values, which counsel us that if you work hard and long enough, you'll be too exhausted to fight with your family. Based on Laura Ingalls Wilder's classic series of childhood memoirs on the great American frontier, *Little House on the Prairie* follows the Ingalls from their home in Wisconsin to their new homestead in Walnut Grove, where they set down their roots and helped build the American heartland, one log at a time. And while the Ingalls ain't got a barrel of money like those uppity Olesons who run the dry-goods store, and they might look ragged and funny, the Ingalls travel along, singing their song, side by side into a Perpetual Syndication Sunrise.

CHAPTER 2

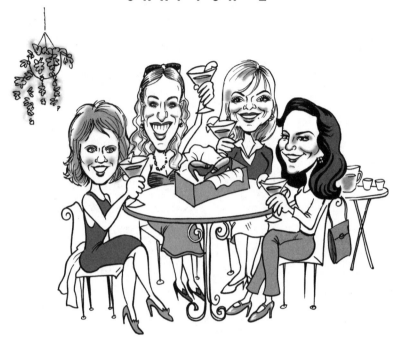

Diva TV

ARE YOU TIRED OF being an extra in the miniseries of your own life? Are you ready to demand your own trailer and bathe in the limelight, only you're too busy making sure that everybody else is getting his fair share of the close-ups? Well, take a Diva TV refresher course in entitlement from some of TV's most notorious queens of control, who hold on to their place in the spotlight by taking hold of themselves, and learn from the best how to take charge of your own remote control.

- *Sex and the City (1998–2004)*
  Stars: Sarah Jessica Parker, Kim Cattrall, Kristin Davis, Cynthia Nixon

From Darren Star, the creator of *Beverly Hills 90210* and *Melrose Place*, comes a diva-thon featuring four single thirtysomething gal pals searching for true love in the big city, and in the process give us all a crash course in how to be fabulous.

And nobody knows fabulous like Darren Star. His *Sex and the City* girls, Carrie (Sarah Jessica Parker), Samantha (Kim Cattrall), Miranda (Cynthia Nixon), and Charlotte (Kristin Davis), eat and shop, have multiple orgasms, and rush to exciting jobs on Jimmy Choo heels. Then they rush off to ring the opening bell at the stock exchange before rushing off to happy-hour dates, and then rush through exotic dinners so that they can rush off to have multiple orgasms and shop and eat some more.

And in their spare time, the girlfriends meet each other in breezy, low-carb Madison Avenue cafés to kiss and tell over Cosmos with a twist of uptown-girl cynicism, and wonder wistfully when they will finally begin to live happily ever after.

And like many of us modern-day Rapunzels who are beginning to feel the clock ticking on our happy ending, these slightly sadder but wiser gals languish in designer-label la-la land, where the heels, the frocks, and the anonymous sex as a political statement are beginning to lose a little of their luster, and they are beginning to wonder when their fairy tales will come true, until the one day when they just do. These women remind us that happy endings come just when you least expect them and in forms we don't always recognize. But until Mr. Big comes along, the *Sex and the City* girls reassure us that there will always be food, and friends, and a city full of fabulous, to keep us happy in the meantime.

WARNING LABEL

We do have to say that while we totally get that it's a whole lot of fun to watch rich, young, beautiful white girls live out a gay man's version of paradise, only without the show tunes, and while we totally understand that it can be a thrilling and liberating feeling to watch chicks treating sex just as casually and objectively as guys do, we kind of wish that the next time the airwaves strike a blow for the fairer sex, they'd choose characters who reinvent their own new definitions of power and fulfillment and freedom, rather than just emulating the failed, self-indulgent extravagances of men.

TV DIVA DIAMONDS

*The fact is, sometimes it's really hard to walk in a single woman's shoes.
That's why we need really special ones now and then to
make the walk a little more fun.*

*Later that day I got to thinking about relationships. There are those that
open you up to something new and exotic, those that are old and familiar,
and those that bring up lots of questions, those that bring you somewhere
unexpected, those that bring you far from where you started, and those that
bring you back. But the most exciting, challenging, and significant
relationship of all is the one you have with yourself. And if you can find
someone to love the you that you love, well, that's just fabulous.*

★ all quotes from Sarah Jessica Parker as Carrie Bradshaw in *Sex and the City*

TV TIDBITS

The final word spoken in the very last episode of *Sex and the City* was *fabulous.*

The Versace "dress of a thousand layers" that Carrie (Sarah Jessica Parker) wore
in the final episode has a retail price of seventy-nine thousand dollars.

■ *Desperate Housewives (2004–)*
*Stars: Teri Hatcher, Felicity Huffman, Marcia Cross, Eva Longoria,
Nicolette Sheridan*

If you're feeling trapped in a suburban wasteland and are desperate to stir a little forbidden fruit into your daily bread, let the women of Wisteria Lane add a little hot sauce to your recipe, without having to deal with the emotional heartburn in the morning.

This series picks up where *Sex and the City* leaves off and carries us away to a bucolic Stepford, where the girls next door, now wives and mothers, move about their impeccable dream homes, carrying out the time-honored rituals of the suburban good life dressed in flawless couture. Then one day the bubble bursts, leaving Mary Alice Young (Brenda Strong), the most desperate of the desperate housewives, with her brains splattered all over her polished parquet floor. On Wisteria Lane, where even the shrubs are shapely, it seems that a dark secret has been growing beneath the meticulous lawns and Martha Stewart manners, and it is up to Mary Alice's friends to figure out what in the world went wrong with Mary Alice.

The women of Wisteria Lane include Susan (Teri Hatcher), a desperate divorcée and single mom; Lynette (Felicity Huffman), a desperate ex-exec turned stay-at-home mom; Bree (Marcia Cross), a psycho-Martha knockoff searching desperately for perfection in an imperfect world; Gabrielle (Eva Longoria), an ex-model desperately hanging on to the kind of youth that only a lot of money can buy; and Edie (Nicolette Sheridan), the man-eater on the block, who is desperately looking for love in all the wrong places . . . and we do mean *all*. As this band of Cheer moms looks beneath the surface to glimpse the truth about Mary Alice, what they get is a good honest look at themselves, and along with them, we discover that the true definition of a domestic diva is a woman who takes responsibility for her own happily ever after, no matter what the neighbors think.

Food Facials: Cool As a Cucumber

After you've been up raking and hoeing 'til the wee hours with supple-limbed and raven-haired landscapers who are emblematic of the doomed beauty of youth and therefore oblivious to the concept of last call, try out this recipe for a cucumber yogurt facial mask before the ladies' bridge club arrives, and only your gardener will know for sure.

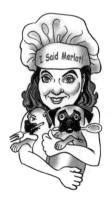

Here's what you'll need:
1 peeled cucumber, sliced
1 tablespoon honey
2 tablespoons plain yogurt
2 big glasses water
Salt, cumin, dill
Pita chips

Here's how you do it:
Puree the peeled cucumber, honey, and yogurt in a blender. Apply half of the cucumber mixture to your face, making sure to leave half in reserve. Keep the mask on for 30 minutes before washing off with cold water. While you wait, pound both glasses of water because you, much like your flower garden, require hydration if you expect the blush to stay on the rose. Season the remaining cucumber mixture with salt, cumin, and dill to taste, and serve with pita chips.

■ *Absolutely Fabulous (1992–)*
Stars: Jennifer Saunders, Joanna Lumley, Julia Sawalha

Nobody defines fabulous quite like Edina and Patsy, two aging blossoms left over from the summer of love, who have been partying like it's 1999 since 1969, with no sign of last call in sight. And what makes *Absolutely Fabulous* such great Diva TV is that despite the perpetually flowing river of vodka and Veuve, the controlled substances, decades of conspicuous consumption, and deplorable interpersonal skills, Eddy and Pats remain the undisputed queens of their realm, because they love each other.

When you're feeling starved for stimulation, Jennifer Saunders's British series, a cult sensation for six seasons and counting, is like a feast of forbidden fabulous. The diva banquet is served up in the Monsoon family kitchen, where sin is in and moderation is a myth, and just about anything goes, as long as it looks and feels good.

Edina Monsoon (Jennifer Saunders) is a blowsy and boozy middle-aged hippie turned nineties-style PR queen who is successful at making everything trendy but herself, and is engaged in an absurd and futile search for what is right under her nose. Forever at her side is her best friend, Patsy Stone (Joanna Lumley), a Twiggy-inspired former model who hasn't eaten or smiled since 1973, and who is at this point held together with Botox and bobby pins. Patsy's inner world can be summed up at any given moment by the height of her blond bouffant, and she lives her life on the verge of an overdose, or at the very least a multiple fracture. And then there's Eddy's daughter, Saffron (Julia Sawalha), the perpetually put-upon foil, who longs for their attention and approval but can't stand either one of them.

In six seasons, Eddy and Pats have managed to violate just about every rule of social acceptability and decorum. And the best part is that these fading glimmer twins don't seem to care. Perhaps it's because they have no consciences, no empathy, and no liver. But maybe too it's because Eddy and Pats have no regrets. Their lives are a pure and accurate expression of themselves. They live without restraint and they calls 'em like they sees 'em, with no apologies.

While we can't say that Edina and Patsy's search for eternal youth will work outside of TV-land, we can tell you that spending a few hours with these lovable divas of excess will kick up the juice on your joie de vivre. Eddy and Pats remind us that being a diva means being brave enough to be your fabulous self and have a fabulous best friend who adores you even when you aren't feeling quite so fabulous.

TV DIVA DIAMONDS

Edina: You-you just sit there like you're velcroed to some bloody adman! You know those crap-head admen over there, you know, those kings of bastardization that have just taken everything that was ever real and genuine and honest and original and attached it to a toilet cleaner! Whereas I-I...like a bird on a wire...like a drunk in a midnight choir... I have tried in my way to be free.

Patsy: Go for it, Eddy.

★ Jennifer Saunders as Edina and Joanna Lumley as Patsy in *Absolutely Fabulous*

CHICKS THAT KICK

Here are some of our favorite female warriors who aren't afraid to kick ass and take names.

Saturday Night Live: The Best of Molly Shannon

Molly Shannon is definitely the chick with kick, and this "best of" captures every step ball change in Molly's repertoire. When she's not kickin' and stretchin' and kickin', she's smellin' her pits and falling into basically everything and reminding us in the process that as long as you've got legs, you can step up to the plate and swing for the bleachers. Her morphing into Courtney Love and Liza is truly hysterical and we're so glad they included the bonus features of her on *Conan*.

Buffy the Vampire Slayer

Sarah Michelle Gellar is one of our favorite teen beat gals who's got legs and knows how to use them. After Buffy burns down her high school gym, she's forced to go to a new school and start her new life as the "chosen one, the Slayer." Buffy, with a little help from her friends, must fight vampires, demons, and the forces of evil while still managing to look like she walked straight off the *Clueless* set. Buffy is a debutante with a difference who proves with each episode and stage-combat class that style is just as important as substance when it comes to fighting the forces of darkness.

Wonder Woman

Wonder Woman (Lynda Carter) is sent by the Amazons to help with the war crisis. Armed with a magic belt, bullet-stopping bracelets, the most dangerous tiara east of West Hollywood, and the most lethal bra this side of Madonna's Blonde Ambition tour, Wonder Woman spins into action and gives evil a swift kick in the rear. Wonder Woman was an alpha chick for the seventies who really knew how to turn it on and turn it out, and still come away looking, well, kinda cheesy. But, hey, it was the seventies, and it's not easy to accessorize a red, white, and blue onesie and go-go boots.

Xena: Warrior Princess

Xena (Lucy Lawless), the mighty female warrior who polices the periphery of the TV outback in search of scoundrels willing to make her day, is like a female Clint Eastwood, only dressed in a faux fur ensemble straight out of a Ringo Starr vehicle, and with distinct homoerotic undertones. And then again, maybe Xena isn't such a departure from the Eastwood brand of heroics after all. Together with her lipstick "companion" Gabrielle (Renée O'Connor), they maintain the purity of their love-free zone, eschewing all admirers, because they are committed to a compulsive effort to assuage Xena's feelings of original guilt. Xena is a warrior princess so haunted by guilt over her bloody past as a continent conqueror that she vows to use all the weapons in her arsenal, including her steely-eyed gaze, her war whoop, and her leather push-up bra, to do good, rather than evil. Xena, who spends her TV life compulsively opening up a can of syndication-worthy whup-ass to compensate for her feelings of unlovability, gets our vote as the mythic embodiment of Freudian theory with the biggest kick.

▪ *The Nanny (1993–1999)*
Stars: Fran Drescher, Daniel Davis, Charles Shaughnessy, Lauren Lane,
    Benjamin Salisbury, Nicholle Tom, Madeline Zima, Renee Taylor,
    Ann Morgan Guilbert, Rachel Chagall

She was workin' at a bridal shop in Flushing, Queens, and as we all now know from the theme song, that's how she became the Nanny.

Fran Fine (Fran Drescher) is a diva from the wrong side of the tracks with big hair and big dreams to match. In fact, the only thing that isn't big is her budget. She happens upon Maxwell Sheffield (Charles Shaughnessy) and lands a job on the right side of Park Avenue. Next thing Fran knows she's running the household, solving problems that are bigger than her bouffant, and falling in love with the man of the house. Also keeping us laughing are Niles, the butler (Daniel Davis), and Mr. Sheffield's business partner, C. C. Babcock

(Lauren Lane). Then, once you throw in Fran's mother and grandmother, we're talking about a *lot* of big hair and *a lot* of kvetching.

Fran is one of our favorite TV divas because while she doesn't bring home the bacon, and certainly never cooks anything up in a pan, she still manages to do a good job raising a family with the most important tool at a diva's disposal: a good sense of humor.

DUELING DIVAS

There's nothing quite like a catfight between a couple of world-class TV bitch goddesses to remind us that no matter how fabulous, no diva is an island, and though you may have creative control, you still have to be nice to your costars.

Karen and Jack in *Will & Grace*

Karen Walker (Megan Mullaly), a pill-popping, martini-swigging, wisecracking widow of a fat man with millions, and Jack McFarland (Sean Hayes), a J-Lo-loving, man-grabbing, disco-dancing legend in his own mind, came together on *Will & Grace* and quickly became one of the most lovable diva duos in TV history. Karen is a little bit Mame and a little bit Anna Nicole, all tucked into the same tailored Bergdorf ensemble, and her best friend, Jack, is like Cher meets Gilligan. And despite the most irresponsible pharmacist in network television and the worst cabaret show in all of the West Village, Karen and Jack still manage to walk that thin line between beast and beauty without falling off their heels, because they are holding hands.

Alexis and Krystle in *Dynasty*

The creators of *Dynasty* took the embodiment of everybody's worst nightmares about a scorned woman, dressed her up in Halston couture, draped a few Harry Winstons around the pressure points, and hit the prime-time jackpot. And an eighties America, trying to tiptoe along the precipice of penury in a pair of platform boogie shoes, relished every over-the-top, chrome-and-glass moment.

Oil tycoon Blake Carrington's (John Forsythe) ex-wife, Alexis (Joan Collins), became one of the campiest and most beloved bitch goddesses ever to strut, stagger, skulk, slug, and scheme her way into the family rooms of America. In fact, Alexis was so popular that *Dynasty* became known as Joan & Co., and Alexis's picture still appears in the pop culture dictionary, cross-referenced under glamour slut and tulle power suit. But Alexis might have gone completely unnoticed were it not for her nemesis, the current Mrs. Got Rocks, Krystle Carrington (Linda Evans), who is the flip side of Alexis's coin, the Madonna to Alexis's whore. Krystle's unyielding blonde helmet of unimpeachable legitimacy and wifely virtue, not to mention those shoulder pads and the startling abundance of silver lamé, made both ends of the double standard look far more dramatic by comparison, and catapulted this duo of dueling divas way up over the top, into the firmament of mythic and timeless TV bitch goddesses we love to hate. And then, of course, there was that mud-wrestling scene.

Amanda and Alison in *Melrose Place*

What could be better than watching the head cheerleader you loved to hate, all grown up and competing in the homecoming queen pageant of the adult world—an ad agency—and winning the CEO crown only to be covered in a bucket full of stage blood?

Amanda Woodward (Heather Locklear, who else?) is blonde, perky, popular, sociopathic, and looks like she was born in a miniskirt with a pair of pom-poms in her hand. Amanda, like Alexis before her, came onto the scene midway through the series and beat those Nielsen ratings into submission with her irrepressible and impeccably tailored badness. But where would Amanda have been without Alison (Courtney Thorne-Smith) to kick around? Alison, the good girl next door, the perpetual president of the student council, was like an exclamation point in the sentence of Amanda's no-one-can-eat-just-one nastiness, and made *Melrose Place*'s number-one girl with the curl right in the middle of her forehead not only bad but deliciously horrid.

EIGHT KAREN DIAMONDS

Grace, I know what guilt is. It's one of those touchy-feely words that people throw around that don't really mean anything.... You know, like "maternal" or "addiction."

Oh, kids ruin everything. I mean, look at the stitching on this. You cannot trust a ten-year-old to do a good hidden button.

Husbands come and go, but the Chanel sling-backs are for life.

They're trying to turn gay people straight. Do they have any idea what this will do to the fall line?

It's Christmas, for goodness' sake. Think about the baby Jesus: up in that tower, letting his hair down...so that the three wise men can climb up and spin the dreidel and see if there are six more weeks of winter.

Okay, rule number one. Unless you're served in a frosted glass, never come within four feet of my lips.

I'm not good or real...I'm evil and imaginary.

Gosh, I don't think that I've ever been stressed out. Why would I be? I've got practically no responsibilities, my job's a breeze, and I've got a killer rack. Good morning!

★ all quotes from Megan Mullally as Karen Walker in *Will & Grace*

Bev's TV Tray: Glamour with a Can Opener Picnic

(Serves you and a couple of nonunion extras)

There's nothing like an afternoon in the great outdoors to put a smile back on the face of even the most exotic and delicate hothouse diva. After all, divas can't live on heated pools and central air alone. Sometimes a girl just needs a little fresh air and a walk in the woods to restore her perspective and prevent emotional mildew.

Fortunately, we divas can be just as fabulous in the great outdoors as we are in our climate-controlled boudoirs as long as we're properly equipped. So go ahead, take a walk in the wild, and bring along this Glamour with a Can Opener Picnic, because when it comes to getting back to nature, a diva should always be prepared.

Ingredients List for the Houseboy

Give this list to your houseboy and send him to the closest gourmet grocery. Tell him to be quick about it or you'll miss the flattering afternoon light.

1. 1 pound truffle mousse pâté (and tell him for God's sake get a thick slice from the middle this time instead of that crusty end cut)
2. Various cans of really expensive and preferably imported delicacies
3. 1 pound St. André cheese or some other triple-cream variety (and tell him for God's sake pick out a chunk that's ripe this time)
4. 1 ounce each of Ossetra, Beluga, or Sevruga caviar
5. Grapes (peeled)
6. Water crackers and toast points
7. 1 bottle of fine imported champagne; okay, 2 bottles, just in case you run into a thirsty park ranger or two (and tell the houseboy for God's sake to make sure the champagne is pink this time and chilled)

When the houseboy returns, check the purchases to make sure that the cheese is ripe, the pink champagne is cold, and the truffle mousse is moist. If it isn't, send him packing, because this is the second time in a row he's brought you warm bubbly and that simply will not do. If everything is as you want it, tell him to assemble the following outdoor essentials on your checklist.

GETTING BACK TO NATURE CHECKLIST
FOR DIVAS DINING AL FRESCO

- Can opener
- Wine bucket
- Houseboy
- China place settings for two
- Stylish folding table and chairs
- Hand-forged sterling silver cheese knife
- Hand-forged mother-of-pearl caviar spoon
- Portable generator
- Extension cord
- Ambient mood lighting
- A gramophone so you can reenact that really romantic safari scene from *Out of Africa*
- Two crystal champagne flutes
- Portable litter and chaise with four well-muscled attendants to bear you aloft
- Peacock feather fan
- A guy in a sarong to wave the peacock feather fan
- Another guy in a sarong to feed you peeled grapes
- A cell phone to call for delivery in case you forgot anything
- Ice

Check your list, check it twice, and tell the houseboy to pack the whole lot to go. Then tell the driver to bring the car around, and start off in the direction of the nearest trailhead. And tell him for God's sake to step on it because you've got reservations in town at eight and you've got to change for dinner, and the maître d' gets huffy when you're late.

When you reach the summit of your breathless peak, tell your houseboy to set up the chaise, break out the can opener, and crack open a bottle of that bubbly. And tell him to be quick about it for God's sake. Then sip a little champagne, nibble a few really expensive and preferably imported delicacies, and get in touch with the beauty and simplicity of nature.

REALITY CHECK

Of course, for us divas who are in between comebacks and are temporarily on a budget, all you really need to refresh your diva spirit and renew your sense of perspective until your next global simulcast is a picnic basket full of a few of your favorite delicacies and a healthy sense of adventure. Oh, and don't forget the can opener.

DISASTERTHERAPY

Because sometimes watching a diva in the midst of a head-on collision with herself reminds us that no matter what we encounter along life's highway, we will survive.

The Anna Nicole Show (2002–2004)
Stars: Anna Nicole Smith, Daniel Smith, Howard K. Stern, Kim Walther, Sugar Pie

As her theme song will tell you, Anna Anna fabulous Anna, Anna Nicole is *sooooooo* outrageous. And her theme song is right: Anna is outrageous. But Anna is something else too, and that is the je ne sais quoi that makes Anna such great Diva TV for all of us would-be cover models with a plus-size appetite for life.

Anna Nicole is a Teflon diva whom the cutlery of life is powerless to chip. She has endured a small-town Texas upbringing, a ten-year probate battle that she recently lost, bankruptcy, single parenthood, the paparazzi, a strawberry-milk and pickle habit, seventy extra pounds, an ambiguous sexual orientation, and the messiest "natural" high we've ever seen, and held on to her divahood. Anna endures because she has held on to her sense of humor. Well, that and an obviously indulgent pharmacist. So if you've got a bad case of the stuck-in-the-glue blues, let Anna Nicole show you how to turn your bars into stars, Mexia, Texas, style.

OUT OF THE MOUTHS OF BABES

I'm always having a good time; I'm a happy person.

I don't care what sex they are, I just like strippers.

Damn, you need to go to church!

I'm so hungry. Where's the cheese doughnut?

Two thumbs up, and if I had more thumbs, it would be more thumbs up.

My life is a roller coaster, so hold on and enjoy the ride!

I liked myself bigger. I've got too many bones.

★ all quotes from Anna Nicole Smith on *The Anna Nicole Show*

Made-for-TV-Movie Medicine

Martha, Inc. *(2003)*
Stars: Cybill Shepherd, Tim Matheson, Joanna Cassidy, Dorie Barton

Speaking of Teflon divas, this camp classic about lifestyle queen Martha Stewart—who nut-cracks her way to the height of power, only to wind up a poor little rich girl who despite her money has no one to love her because she puts her ambition in front of her family—takes potshots galore at America's favorite domestic goddess but is unable to dent the veneer.

Cybill Shepherd stars as Martha, an ambitious and competent woman driven by some kind of imperfectly drawn father issue to claw her way to the top, without giving a second thought to the wear and tear on the people around her. Martha throws pots at her friends, emasculates her husbands, neglects her child, torments the neighbors, and anyone who gets in her way is trussed up like a turkey and roasted until he's good and done. *Martha, Inc.* is TV's interpretation of the vengeful bitch as camp diva genre that Faye Dunaway created with her performance as Joan Crawford in *Mommie Dearest*, and we guarantee, the utensils really fly. This instant camp classic diva movie reminds us that even if you are the most perfect person in the world, if Cybill Shepherd is cast to play you in the TV movie of your life, it's not gonna be pretty. So if you're in the mood for a dose of the dark side of diva, pop in *Martha Inc.*, and for a few hours only, tell the world that you said *merlot*!

MARTHA'S MOXIE

I can almost bend steel with my mind. I can bend anything if I try hard enough. I can make myself do almost anything. But you can get too strong like that, so you have to be careful. You have to temper your strength.

I think baking cookies is equal to Queen Victoria running an empire.
There's no difference in how seriously you take the job, how seriously you
approach your whole life. That's why when people say, "Are you a
feminist?" I say, "No, I'm not." I believe in a man and a woman being
equal. I really believe that we can do anything we set our minds to.

I probably think more about nature than I think about myself.

I would like to be back [from prison] as early in March as possible to plant
a spring garden and to truly get things growing again.

★ all quotes from Cybill Shepherd as Martha Stewart in *Martha, Inc.*

■ *Dynasty* (1981–1989)
Stars: John Forsythe, Linda Evans, Joan Collins, Pamela Sue Martin, Heather Locklear

This episodic saga focuses on the life and times of the Carringtons, an oil-rich family based in Denver that commits every crime of passion that an energetic team of prime-time soap opera writers could think up. Lives were lost, children nabbed, empires seized, and loves stolen in the Carringtons' luscious living room, viewed through a lens softly, and dripping in white diamonds, black leather, and French lace. Oh, and a lot of mirrors.

But what made this show a Saturday-evening phenom, and set water coolers to boiling across America in the Reagan eighties, was that each week we could always count on a catfight between three divas, who elevated big hair, big jewelry, and big shoulder pads to the level of the divine. What TV fan can resist a show that offers three divas for the price of one?

Alexis Morell Carrington Colby Dexter Rowan (Joan Collins), Krystle Grant Jennings Carrington (Linda Evans), and Samantha Josephine "Sammy Jo" Dean Reece Carrington Fallmont (Heather Locklear) battle it out week in and week out, ostensibly to gain control of the Carrington fortune, but mostly just for the pleasure sport of breaking the nails of the competition. And of course, this was the eighties, so there was always Blake Carrington himself (John Forsythe), the Reagan-esque good husband and father in the background, who controlled the purse strings and wouldn't let these Nancys get too far out of hand. So if you're ready to bust your sequins and are longing to initiate a hostile takeover, spend a few hours in the Carringtons' living room and let Alexis and Krystle and Sammy Jo (not to mention the later entrance of Millie "Dominique" Cox Deveraux [Diahann Carroll]) show you how to build a TV dynasty Denver style, and let the Baccarat fly without waking up with a concussion.

Bev's TV Tray: Fried Men

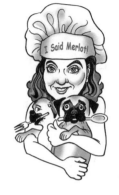

Is your inner pressure cooker approaching critical mass? Before you blow your lid, try out this recipe for Fried Men, because there's nothing like deep-frying somebody in effigy to take the edge off. You can decorate them too. Dress up your men to suggest people who have really been on your nerves lately. Fashion little dough ties, or pastry palm pilots. Give your men little self-satisfied grins, which you can then wipe off their little fried faces. Or make everybody nervous and serve your fried men headless. Go ahead, express yourself! The only limits are the ones imposed by your imagination and your superego.

As with most things in life, really good fried men require a little patience, a firm hand, and a reliable fire extinguisher, just to be on the safe side. But don't worry, with the right degree of punching, kneading, and boiling oil, your fried men will usually fall right into line.

Here's what you'll need:
1 cup lukewarm milk
¼ cup sugar
1 tablespoon salt
1 cake compressed yeast
1 egg
¼ cup shortening
3½ cups flour
Dash nutmeg, allspice, and cinnamon
1 cup canola oil
Powdered sugar
Assorted sprinkles, raisins for decorating

Here's how you do it:

In a large bowl combine the milk, sugar, and salt. Next, crumble the yeast into the mix and stir until it's dissolved. Stir in the egg, shortening, and spices, then add the flour. Knead the dough until it's too beaten down to offer any more resistance, then place in a greased bowl and turn it to bring the greased side up. Cover with a damp towel and let the dough rise in a warm place until it's doubled in bulk (about 1 to 1$\frac{1}{2}$ hours). Your dough should be sticky but workable in your hands.

When the dough has gotten itself all puffed up as men, er, dough is known to do, smack it down with your fist until it's completely deflated. Then let it puff up again, which you know it will, until it's almost twice its original size (about 30 to 45 minutes). Then roll out the dough on a floured board until the dough is $\frac{1}{3}$ inch thick and cut with a gingerbread man cookie cutter. Let your men rise for another 30 to 45 minutes and then heat the oil, throw your men into the frying pan, and let them stay there until you can stick a fork in them and turn them over because they're done. Drain on paper towels and let cool.

To decorate, make a glaze out of two parts powdered sugar and one part water, or use colored sugar, sprinkles, or even raisins to personalize your fried men. Then drown them in honey, syrup, or maple cream and macerate them, one limb at a time.

GUY DIVAS

Because what's good for the goose is good for the gander.

Dallas (1978–1991)

Stars: Larry Hagman, Barbara Bel Geddes, Patrick Duffy, Linda Gray, Victoria Principal, Charlene Tilton, Ken Kerchaval, Jim Davis

Never was there a guy diva with a bigger hat than J. R. Ewing (Larry Hagman), who ran his daddy's ranch (a daddy, mind you, whose name was *Jock Ewing*) and his daddy's Dallas-based oil empire like a private fiefdom, and never let anybody sneak up on him from behind, except only that once. Of course, this didn't stop good brother Bobby (Patrick Duffy), or his former-Miss-Texas and money-grubbing wife Sue Ellen (Linda Gray), or the Mary Anne on J. R. Ewing's uncharted desert isle, Pamela (Victoria Principal), from trying to blow his lid off each and every time they got a good, clear shot. Watching J. R. in action is like a crash course in good old boydom, and establishes once and for all that divas don't always come in spike heels and sequined gowns. Sometimes they wear cowboy boots and really bad Western-cut leisure suits and ten-gallon Stetsons.

J.R. GEMS

Barnes just broke the cardinal rule in politics: never get caught in bed with a dead woman or a live man.

Ray never was comfortable eating with the family; we do use knives and forks.

Lots of men have tried to run roughshod over me. You can visit them in the cemetery.

Say, why don't you have that junior plastic surgeon you married design you a new face: one without a mouth!

A marriage is like a salad: the man has to know how to keep his tomatoes on the top.

Cliff, sharpen up your ice skates; it's gonna be a long winter.

Don't forgive and never forget; do unto others before they do unto you; and third and most importantly, keep your eye on your friends, because your enemies will take care of themselves.

★ all quotes from Larry Hagman as J. R. Ewing in *Dallas*

Frasier *(1993–2004)*
*Stars: Kelsey Grammer, David Hyde Pierce, John
Mahoney, Jane Leeves, Peri Gilpin, Moose*

Dr. Frasier Crane leaves his broken marriage, not to mention a
legendary and long-running hit TV series (*Cheers*), to move to Seattle into
his own apartment, his own radio talk show, and, we imagine, his own
dressing room, and proves that even a balding egghead with a taste for
Elizabethan literature, obscure Bach fugues, stinky cheese, and Freud can
be a diva, as long as he gets good enough ratings.

Dr. Crane (Kelsey Grammer) is joined in his midlife search for personal
fulfillment by his ex-cop dad (John Mahoney), who comes complete with
his dog, Eddie (Moose), his physical therapist, Daphne (Jane Leeves), and
possibly one of the ugliest recliners ever seen on TV. And while Frasier
may fall perpetually short of his own legendary vision of himself, he does
manage to remind us all that education, culture, and good old-fashioned
brain-power really can be fabulous in the right light.

DIVA DIAMONDS

*You don't understand. It's not the same as Dad being wrong, or your being
wrong. I have a degree from Harvard. Whenever I'm wrong,
the world makes a little less sense.*

*By tonight my dad will be safely back in his beer-stained, flea-infested,
duct-taped recliner, adjusting his shorts with one hand and cheering on
Jean-Claude Van Damme with the other. Yes, it's quite a little piece
of heaven I've carved out for myself, isn't it?*

I like your self-assurance. There's no greater aphrodisiac than confidence.

I know how bleak these times can be, but believe me, they will come to an end sometime or later. I remember a time back in Boston; I was going through exactly what you're going through now. Just a week later I met a lovely barmaid, sophisticated if a bit loquacious. We fell madly in love and we got engaged.... 'Course, she left me standing at the altar. But the point is, I didn't give up. I took my poor battered heart and handed it to Lilith... who put it in her little Cuisinart and hit the puree button. But I rebounded! And look how far I've come. I'm divorced, lonely, and living with my father.

★ all quotes by Kelsey Grammer as Frasier in *Frasier*

LIVE TO TAPE

Lisa Kudrow was originally cast as Roz but was replaced before production began.

The show's theme song, "Tossed Salad and Scrambled Eggs," was performed by Kelsey Grammer.

Frasier has won more Emmys than any other show in TV history.

After *Cheers* had finished filming, the bar was taken down and the *Frasier* sets were built over it.

Jason's Minibar—The Divatini

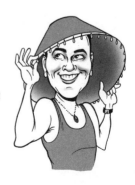

When you're watching one of your favorite divas burn things off with this fabulous divatini that's guaranteed provided you don't exhale too close to an open flame.

Here's what you'll need:
A shaker and lots of ice
Vermouth
A bottle of your favorite vodka
Green olives

Here's how you do it:
Place your martini glasses in the freezer while you're preparing the drink. Fill your shaker with ice to the very top and add a small splash of vermouth. Fill the rest with vodka (and olive juice if you're feeling down and dirty) and then shake-shake-shake until your vodka is good and chilled. Next, retrieve your frosted martini glasses from the freezer, plop in the olives, and pour your divatini over the olives all the way up to the brim. Then toast yourself and sip while you plot your next cliff-hanger.

CHAPTER 3

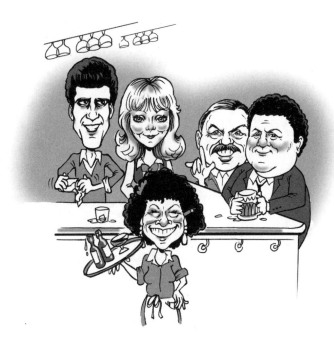

You've Got a Friend TV

WHETHER IT'S JUST YOU and your remote control, home alone feeling bitter, bored, bloated, and blue, or you're in the mood to invite a few friends over and celebrate your bond, serve up a double scoop of You've Got a Friend TV, featuring some of TV's best friends, and be reminded that as long as you've got love in your heart, a relatively decent coffee bar somewhere in town populated with beautiful, upwardly mobile, and surprisingly witty starlets just like you, ice cream, and reliable cable service, you're never really alone.

■ *Seinfeld (1990–1998)*
Stars: Jerry Seinfeld, Julia Louis-Dreyfus, Michael Richards, Jason Alexander

The father of all friends shows, *Seinfeld* features a group of thirtysomething New York pals who spend most of their time sweating the small stuff together. And in *Seinfeld* world, it's *all* small stuff. Birth, death, love, war, employment, and random street crime are served up as a side dish to the real main events of life, like dropping your toothbrush in the toilet, losing your car in a parking garage, finding the perfect chocolate babka, or seeing Elaine's nipple. As Jerry (Jerry Seinfeld), his ex-girlfriend turned bosom buddy Elaine (Julia Louis-Dreyfus), the thoroughly unredeemable George (Jason Alexander), and the emotional ex-traterrestrial and double-jointed Kramer (Michael Richards) make their way, hand in hand, through the hilariously absurd trivia of everyday life, we begin to understand that life really is what happens while you're circling the airport, but life in a holding pattern isn't so bad, so long as you're sitting in the friendship seat, surrounded by the people who love you.

SEINFELD'S SMALL STUFF

You see, Elaine, the key to eating a black-and-white cookie is that you wanna get some black and some white in each bite. Nothing mixes better than vanilla and chocolate. And yet still somehow racial harmony eludes us. If people would only look to the cookie, all our problems would be solved.
★ Jerry Seinfeld in *Seinfeld*

When she threw that toupee out the window, it was the best thing that ever happened to me. I feel like my old self again. Neurotic, paranoid, totally inadequate, completely insecure. It's a pleasure.
★ Jason Alexander as George Costanza in *Seinfeld*

You know, Darren, if you would have told me twenty-five years ago that someday I'd be standing here about to solve the world's energy problems, I would've said you're crazy....Now let's push this giant ball of oil out the window.
★ Michael Richards as Cosmo Kramer in *Seinfeld*

Why does Radio Shack ask for your phone number when you buy
batteries? I don't know.
★ Michael Richards as Cosmo Kramer in *Seinfeld*

I met this lawyer, we went out to dinner, I had the lobster bisque, we went
back to my place, yada yada yada, I never heard from him again.
★ Julia Louis-Dreyfus as Elaine Benes in *Seinfeld*

▪ *Friends (1994–2004)*
Stars: Lisa Kudrow, Jennifer Aniston, Courteney Cox, Matthew Perry,
  Matt LeBlanc, David Schwimmer

What do you get when you combine six friends, one apartment building, and the Big Apple in prime time? Well, in the case of these famous friends, you get a decade of laughs, tears, struggles, love, loss, and a great reminder that there's nothing in life that you can't get through, with a little help from your friends.

Rachel (Jennifer Aniston), Monica (Courteney Cox), Phoebe (Lisa Kudrow), Joey (Matt LeBlanc), Chandler (Matthew Perry), and Ross (David Schwimmer) are all young adults fresh off the boat with big dreams and no clues. The characters are archetypal and relatively indicative of any group of twentysomethings these days: there's the lovable blonde ditz, the geek with the soul of a champion, the meathead with the dazzling smile, and of course, the tramp with a heart of gold. The group hangs out (and some characters at times even work) at Central Perk, the boob tube's interpretation of Starbucks, which was the social hub of the era.

But the dilemmas that these characters confront in each episode are far from house blend. From Chandler's tranny dad (Kathleen Turner), to Phoebe finding a human thumb in her soda can, to Joey playing Al Pacino's butt double, crazy things happen to this freakishly normal group of kids, and somehow, with the help of the bond between them, they manage to prevail and stumble their way into adulthood together, which is a good thing, as most of them were well into their thirties by the time the show finally ended.

So when you and your friends are struggling with the cataclysmic banality of growing up, watch this support group of a sitcom and remember that no matter what time slot you wind up in on the network of your life, *Friends* will always be on somewhere.

FRIEND FACTS

During two years of its run, *Friends* was filmed on the same soundstage as *Full House*.

The first member of the *Friends* cast to get a role in a Hollywood film was actually Marcel (Ross's pet monkey).

The first love interest was originally going to be between Joey and Monica.

Courteney Cox was asked to play Rachel, but after reading the parts she asked to play Monica.

Across the Hall, *Friends Like Us*, *Insomnia Café*, and *Six of One* were all titles considered before it was decided the show would be called *Friends*.

Central Perk is a real café in NYC's West Village.

Téa Leoni was first offered the part of Monica, but she turned it down.

The final episode of *Friends* aired on May 6, 2004, to an audience of 51.1 million people.

▪ *The Mary Tyler Moore Show* (1970–1977)
  Stars: *Mary Tyler Moore, Edward Asner, Gavin McLeod,*
    Valerie Harper, Ted Knight, Cloris Leachman

Mary Tyler Moore stars as Mary Richards, one of TV's very first single career gals, who comes to the big city all alone after a bad breakup, with no particular plan in mind, and winds up becoming the first woman in network television to understand that it's friends that make a family.

The Mary Tyler Moore Show introduced a new American dream for all of us who felt hemmed in by small-town romance and small-town dreams, but worried about winding up lost in the valley of the dolls all by ourselves if we ventured out alone after dark. Mary Richards reassured us that establishing our independence didn't have to mean that we would wind up alone. Maybe we'd wind up like Mary—living in a charming loft on the second floor of a quaint old Victorian in a friendly city. Maybe we would make friends that felt just like family and find a job that we really cared about. Maybe we, like Mary, could make it after all. It is no wonder that the *Mary Tyler Moore* theme song is the number-one requested birthday anthem in downtown piano bars that specialize in such things.

So if you're wondering how you're going to make it on your own, and just in the mood to turn a nothing day into something that somehow seems worthwhile, spend a few hours with Mary and the gang, who remind us that love is all around, so there's no need to waste it, and that we have the time, if we would only take it.

MARY MOMENTS

I get to thinking that my job is too important to me. And I tell myself that the people I work with are just the people I work with. But last night I thought what is family anyway? It's the people who make you feel less alone and really loved.
★ Mary Tyler Moore as Mary Richards in *The Mary Tyler Moore Show*

No, Mare, cottage cheese solves nothing; chocolate can do it all!
★ Valerie Harper as Rhoda Morgenstern in *The Mary Tyler Moore Show*

I'm an experienced woman. I've been around.... Well, all right, I might not've been around, but I've been...nearby.
★ Mary Tyler Moore as Mary Richards in *The Mary Tyler Moore Show*

I was lying in bed last night and I couldn't sleep, and I came up with an idea. So I went right home and wrote it down.
★ Betty White as Sue Ann Nivens in *The Mary Tyler Moore Show*

TV TIDBITS

The show was originally planned to be about a divorced woman, but because divorce was still a hot subject in 1970, they settled for a broken engagement instead. Also, the network was afraid people would think that Mary had divorced Rob Petrie, the husband of her character on *The Dick Van Dyke Show*, losing the audience's sympathy. After several seasons, the theme song was completely rewritten and the last line went from "you might just make it after all" to "you're gonna make it after all."

■ *Melrose Place (1992–1999)*
Stars: *Thomas Calabro, Josie Bissett, Heather Locklear, Andrew Shue, Jack Wagner, Grant Show, Daphne Zuniga, Doug Savant, Courtney Thorne-Smith, Marcia Cross, Laura Leighton*

Melrose Place focuses on the lives and loves of a group of twentysomethings who all live in the same apartment complex called Melrose Place, and who remind us that even if your closest compatriots try to steal your wife or take your life, in the end you can all still be friends, just as long as you can pay the rent.

Michael (Thomas Calabro), Jane (Josie Bissett), Billy (Andrew Shue), Jake (Grant Show), Peter (Jack Wagner), Jo Beth (Daphne Zuniga), Matt (Doug Savant), Allison (Courtney Thorne-Smith), Kimberly (Marcia Cross), and Sydney (Laura Leighton) are an incestuous group of young professionals who play out their lives and loves all under one roof. Originally the conflicts between these young, beautiful, and upwardly mobile friends and neighbors picked up where *Beverly Hills 90210* left off. But by midseries, as ratings flagged, executive producer Aaron Spelling called in the evil sorceress Amanda (Heather Locklear), who clip-clopped in on impossibly high pumps, wearing a miniskirt and a senior veep title, and started messing with everybody's billing. And before we could click our heels, we weren't in West Hollywood anymore—we were in Falcon Crest. Soon babies were being snatched, hardworking employees were sacked, loves were lost, and hearts were broken.

Yet despite Sydney's pyromania, Jane's paralysis, Michael's felonious infidelity, and Matt's serostatus, everybody winds up friends in the end. Even with Amanda. Of course, the apartment complex itself didn't prove quite as resilient as the bricks and mortar of friendship.

So if you're feeling all on your lonesome, and like you haven't got a friend in the world, peer through the windows of *Melrose Place* and vicariously experience the thrills and spills of extreme friendship, which you would never, ever want to live through firsthand, and be thankful that you're home safe on your couch in Kansas.

ETERNAL QUESTIONS

Matt: How can you stay with a woman who tried to kill you?
Michael: Do I judge your lifestyle, Matt?
★ Doug Savant as Matt and Thomas Calabro as Michael in *Melrose Place*

Are we working? Or are you gonna mate right in front of me?
★ Alyssa Milano as Jennifer Mancini in *Melrose Place*

Divorced, married, widowed, and all in, what, forty-eight hours?
★ Heather Locklear as Amanda in *Melrose Place*

Is your memory that selective or are you just suffering from some grand delusion?
★ Heather Locklear as Amanda in *Melrose Place*

By the way, Kimberly, how is electroshock going?
★ Laura Leighton as Sydney in *Melrose Place*

BAD HAIR DAY TV

If you've just washed your hair and you can't do a thing with it, and you're in need of a little emotional conditioning, tune in to some Bad Hair Day TV and be reminded that the best makeovers work from the inside out, because even supermodels sometimes feel fat.

America's Next Top Model (2003–)

Tyra Banks hosts this competition to see who is going to be America's next superstar cover girl. Beautiful hopefuls are selected to compete in a rigorous competition for the limelight. To gain the brass ring, these contestants must not only be beautiful, but must also be able to do stuff like pose with poisonous spiders, inhabit a tortured gay designer's vision of their personal alter ego without looking frightened on film, and most important, learn how to stay the hell out of Tyra's limelight. As they struggle to outmodel each other for the top slot, these high-fashion beauty queens, who live in close quarters with the competition, scratch and strut among themselves and wind up learning along with the rest of us that feeling beautiful has nothing to do with what we look like on the outside, but how we feel on the inside.

Queer Eye for the Straight Guy (2003–)
Stars: Kyan Douglas, Ted Allen, Jai Rodriguez, Thom Filicia, Carson Kressley

Five gay men team up to transform domestically, aesthetically, and romantically challenged straight guys into metrosexual leading men who can discuss their feelings, open a bottle of wine without using their teeth, and aren't afraid to admit they had a facial. In the spirit of *Charlie's Angels*, Carson, Kyan, Ted, Thom, and Jai barge in, curling wands drawn, dispensing advice on everything from food to fashion to personal hygiene. In the course of just one hour, they turn stuffy into sumptuous, cramped into camp, and remind all of us in the process that the best accessory in any fashion arsenal is self-confidence. So if you're in the midst of a male-pattern balding day, let the Fab

Five remind you that the only difference between a prince and a frog is a secure self-image, a fatherly shoulder to lean on, and the gender confidence to use a little product now and again when you've got a bad case of split ends.

Celebrity Fit Club (2002–)

If you're in the midst of a water-retention moment, there is nothing more comforting than watching celebrities who are way fatter than you feel, trying to do calisthenics and just say no to Twinkies, and failing on national TV. Where else can you find a Baldwin gone to bloat, Liv Tyler's pudgy sister, *Divorce Court's* Judge Mablean in spaghetti straps, *and* Biz Markie with his pants down all on one TV show? This show is like Trim Spa for the soul.

Bev's TV Tray: Be Your Own Best Friend Fries

There's nothing like a little beige food when you're feeling khaki, and there's nothing khakier than french fries. In order to enjoy the full benefits of this comfort food, however, the first thing you have to do is to disconnect the hard wiring that pushes the guilt button every time you sit down to a few thousand empty calories.

So before you begin deep frying, sit down, take a deep cleansing breath, disconnect from the intergenerational chain of culinary conflicts, and tell yourself that french fries are only a potato. Whether golden, crinkled, shoe-stringed, waffle cut, or curly, french fries have been making people from Ashtabula to Tucumcari feel better after a bad day for centuries. And besides, if it weren't for french fries, how would a cheeseburger ever become deluxe?

Here's what you'll need:

> Idaho or russet potatoes (as many as you can manage to slice without flirting
>   with carpal tunnel syndrome—say 3 to 4 large, peeled)
>
> 4 tablespoons powdered sugar
>
> 2 cups vegetable oil
>
> A lot of salt
>
> A lot of ketchup

Here's how you do it:

> As with most things in life, there's more than one way to cut a fry. I usually cut
> the potatoes into ½- to ¾-inch slabs and then cut the slabs again into ½-inch strips.
> There's room for some individual creative expression here, which is a good thing, as
> french fries make me feel expansive and lyrical.
>
> Next, dissolve the powdered sugar in 4 cups water, and soak your sliced potatoes
> in the sugar water until you just can't wait any longer. But try to hold out for at least
> 10 to 15 minutes, because it really does make a difference. Then drain the potatoes.
> Heat your oil in a frying pan at least six inches deep until the oil is hot. When you
> think it's hot enough, toss in enough fries to allow them to swim around a little bit.
> In fact, as with most things, it's a good idea to encourage them to swim rather than
> sink. When your fries are the appropriate shade of golden brown, dump them out
> onto paper towels, salt generously, slather with ketchup, and serve immediately.

▪ *Cheers* (1982–1993)
Stars: Ted Danson, Shelley Long, Kirstie Alley, Nicholas Colasanto,
  Rhea Perlman, Woody Harrelson, Kelsey Grammer, Bebe Neuwirth,
  John Ratzenberger, George Wendt

If you want to go someplace where everybody knows your name, stop in and bend an elbow with the gang at *Cheers*, and experience the camaraderie that only good friends and cold beer can bring, without having to face the hangover in the morning.

Sam "Mayday" Malone (Ted Danson), a former star baseball player who has a problem with the broads and the booze, decides to give up the bottle and open a bar (good thinking,

Sam) in Boston. Before he knows it, his pub, which is called Cheers, becomes home plate for a jeery and beery gang of characters who find comfort, friendship, and laughter at Sam's friendly neighborhood watering hole.

The *Cheers* gang includes Diane Chambers (Shelley Long), an aspiring novelist/waitress who falls in and out of love with Sam at least twice in every episode. There's Carla (Rhea Perlman), the perpetually pregnant waitress who serves up her brew with a snarl and a sassy one-liner, Woody (Woody Harrelson), the small-town boy with an empty head and a heart of gold, Cliff (John Ratzenberger), the postal postman, and Norm (George Wendt), the hard-drinking, softhearted barfly who lives for his friends, his offstage wife, and one more pull of the beer tap. And, as there is always one in every crowd, *Cheers* has a resident neurotic. Dr. Frasier Crane (Kelsey Grammer) was the high-strung, pseudosophisticated psychiatrist who so appealed to the anti-intellectual snobbery of the eighties audiences that he spun off into his own hit series.

So when you need a break from the madness that lies outside the tavern doors, stop off for a couple at *Cheers*, and raise a glass to Boston, baseball, beer, and the buddies who get us through the long winter, until our next opening day.

NORM'S BEER NUTS

It's terrorists, Sam. They've taken over my stomach and they're demanding beer.

Women, you can't live with 'em. Pass the beer nuts.

I'm on top of the world…it's a dismal spot in Greenland somewhere.

A thirsty guy walks into a bar…you finish it.

Buy me a pitcher, you can kiss me on the lips.
★ all quotes from George Wendt as Norm in *Cheers*

▪ *Ally McBeal (1997–2002)*
  Stars: Calista Flockhart, Gil Bellows, Greg Germann,
    Courtney Thorne-Smith, Peter MacNicol, Jane Krakowski,
    Lisa Nicole Carson

Ally McBeal, who is a lot like Mary Tyler Moore meets Elle in *Legally Blonde*, is a heroine for all of us disappointed debutantes who are suddenly thrust out all alone into a world we didn't choose. Ally reassures us that while sometimes we don't always get or even want what's best for us, if we listen to life and trust our friends, we'll usually find our way to a happy ending after all.

Ally McBeal (Calista Flockhart) follows her childhood sweetheart, Billy (Gil Bellows), into Harvard Law School, even though she has absolutely no interest whatsoever in law (strike one). When Billy dumps her anyway, she continues to carry a torch for him (strike two). When her school chum hires Ally to work at the same firm that Billy is working at and Ally takes the job (and you're out), Ally is set adrift into a vast and unfriendly sea of tort reform and tortured romance, and just about goes under. But with the love and advice of her friends and colleagues, including her loose-lipped secretary, Elaine (Jane Krakowski), her roommate and resident expert on *affaires du coeur*, Renee (Lisa Nicole Carson), and her nemesis, Georgia (Courtney Thorne-Smith)—plus a really active imagination that regularly leaps out of her head and onto the screen—Ally is able to make it after all. Not only does Ally appeal to anyone who has ever woken up and said, "What am I doing in a law firm?" (and there are a lot of us out there), she also reminds us in the process that life, love, and work are only as good as the quality of our friendships.

ALLY'S LEGAL BRIEFS

We're not only wired to want what we can't have, but we're also wired to want what we really don't want.

When guys are persistent, it's romantic, they make movies about that. If it's a woman, then they cast Glenn Close.

Law and love are the same—romantic in concept but the actual practice can give you a yeast infection.

I like being a mess. It's who I am.

★ all quotes from Calista Flockhart as Ally McBeal in *Ally McBeal*

■ *Thirtysomething (1987–1991)*
  Stars: Ken Olin, Mel Harris, Timothy Busfield, Patricia Wettig, Luke Rossi, Melanie Mayron, Polly Draper, Peter Horton

This prime-time soap opera about a group of thirtysomething friends trying to leave adolescence behind at last and act like grown-ups was a TV attempt to grab hold of the baby boomer generation's hopes and fears, in the same way that *The Big Chill* had, only without Smokey Robinson and his whiter shade of pale.

This TV show gave birth to the idea that watching a group of young adults struggling to embrace their inevitable destiny as upper-middle-class married yuppies with kids, increasingly distant friendships, and a mortgage was actually entertaining. And while this ultrasuburban soap opera could have descended into white wining, the show was held aloft by the same production team that brought us *My So-Called Life*, and remained a sometimes painfully accurate but always loving portrait of the ups and downs of the yuppie years, when we were all trying to grow up and be responsible like our parents, but were resisting the inevitable isolation and terrible loneliness that is at the core of the surreal suburban American dream.

Jason's Minibar—The Friendly Margarita

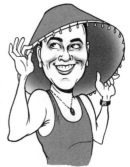

Daisies are the friendliest flower, and this margarita, which is the Spanish word for "daisy," will help you celebrate when you're spending the night in front of the TV with your favorite couch buddies.

Here's what you'll need:
   One bottle of your favorite tequila
   Sweet-and-sour mix (or fresh lime juice mixed with simple syrup)
   Triple sec
   Ice
   Lime wedges

Here's how you do it:

Put one part tequila, one part sweet-and-sour mix, and one part triple sec (about 1½ ounces of each per guest) into the blender and fill with ice to the top. Mix well and pour into margarita or martini glass. Garnish with a lime wedge and enjoy!

CHAPTER 4

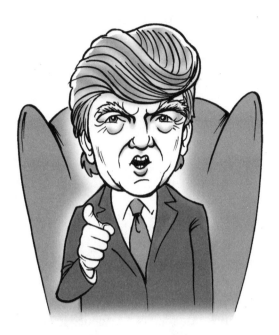

Work Is Hell TV

IF YOU'VE HAD A rough day at the office and you're ready to chuck it all, move to Fiji, and take up shell painting, try unwinding instead with some Work Is Hell TV and watch some other poor schmuck get the pink slip. These shows feature working stiffs just like you and me, who maintain their balance on the steep ladder of success with a good sense of humor, the camaraderie of their colleagues, and a few well-timed commercial breaks. So go ahead, hang up your hard hat, break open the chips, and let somebody else take the lumps for a change while you relax and heal your strained joie de vivre.

▪ *The West Wing* (1999–)
   Stars: *Martin Sheen, Allison Janney, Rob Lowe, Stockard Channing,
      Richard Schiff, Bradley Whitford, John Spencer*

Don't worry, it happens to us all. Every once in a while, we have one of those days when the dog wags us, and no matter how hard we work, no matter how many backs we scratch or hands we wash, or bills we pass, somebody comes up short…and he's not very happy about it. At times like this, spend a few hours in the West Wing and reassure yourself that even the president of the United States has a few tough days at the office and has to call in the relief troops from time to time, to keep the wolves at bay.

The West Wing takes us behind the curtain in a political Oz, and reveals just how many hardworking people it takes to keep the wizard in office and maintain peace and prosperity in the Emerald City.

White House staffers Sam Seaborn (Rob Lowe), C. J. Cregg (Allison Janney), Toby Ziegler (Richard Schiff), Josh Lyman (Bradley Whitford), and Leo McGarry (John Spencer) spend their lives spinning information to make sure that the president can run the country without running afoul of a divided constituency in the volatile world of American government.

At the pinnacle of this political house of cards is President Jeb Bartlett (Martin Sheen), a man of the people who governs from the hip, and as a consequence, often runs afoul of just about every issue-oriented organization and special-interest group in the country. Throw in a few hostile foreign neighbors, a handful of moral conflicts, a voracious press, and a boatload of really pissed-off lobbyists from the other party, and we begin to understand why President Bartlett's staffers drink so much coffee.

We also begin to understand that while we may go off message and take a few lumps from time to time, at least we're not engaged in a perpetual battle with national approval polls in order to ensure our job security.

The West Wing is not only a savvy and sophisticated lesson in the intricacies of politics, but a great reminder that while it's impossible to please all of the people all of the time, if we stay true to our moral compass, hold on to our sense of humor, and find the grace to admit when we're wrong (not to mention maintain a round-the-clock staff of firecracker communication specialists with a flair for metaphor), you really can remain in control of your own personal White House.

HAIL TO THE CHIEF

I was wrong. I was, I was just...I was wrong. No one in government takes responsibility for anything anymore, we fuster, we obfuscate, we rationalize. "Everybody does it," that's what we say. So we come to occupy a moral safe house where everyone's to blame, so no one's guilty. I'm to blame. I was wrong.

"We hold these truths to be self-evident," they said, "that all men are created equal." Strange as it may seem, that was the first time in history that anyone had ever bothered to write that down. Decisions are made by those who show up.

I got an intelligence briefing, a security briefing, and a ninety-minute budget meeting all scheduled for the same forty-five minutes. Are you sure this is a good time to talk about my sense of humor?

I want to call senators. Start with our friends; when we're done with those two, we'll go on to the other ninety-eight.

Can we get this godforsaken event over with so I can get back to presiding over a civilization gone to hell in a handcart?

If I cook the stuffing inside my turkey, can I kill my guests? I'm not saying that would be a deal breaker.

★ all quotes from Martin Sheen as President Jeb Bartlett in *The West Wing*

Bev's TV Tray: Bipartisan Chicken

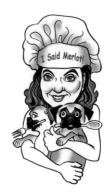

When you're having rival delegates over for dinner, you might want to consider whipping up this impressive meal to secure the peace. This is one of the most delicious dishes ever created through the deft wielding of a meat mallet, and just goes to show you the magnificent results that can ensue from a little creative punishment. Plus, the cathartic relief you'll discover from swinging a meat bat around for a few minutes will do wonders for your stress level. Let's face it: pounding meat is good for you.

Here's what you'll need:
4 boneless and skinless chicken breasts
1 cup flour
4 tablespoons butter
Juice of 2 lemons
2 tablespoons capers
Salt and pepper to taste

Here's how you do it:
Put your chicken breasts, one at a time, into a gallon-size plastic zippered bag and lay flat. Then grab your meat mallet and pound the hell out of it using first the textured side and then the flat side of your mallet. Go ahead, let it all out. Then turn it over and do the other side. When your chicken is thin and flat, and incapable of launching an insurrection, exchange it for another and pound that one too. And then do it again. And again.

Next, coat the chicken in flour. In a large skillet, melt the butter over medium heat and brown the chicken cutlets on both sides until they're golden. Then add lemon juice and capers, cover, and simmer until they're no longer pink and the juice runs clear (about 15 to 20 minutes). Season with salt and pepper to taste.

DISASTER THERAPY

Because sometimes every working stiff needs to watch a good old-fashioned TV train wreck to remind us how fabulous we are by comparison.

The Simple Life (2003–)

Paris Hilton and Nicole Richie are spoiled rich girls who pack it up and take it on the road into small-town middle-class America, where the rules, the houses, and most important, the bank balances, are not at all what Paris and Nicole are accustomed to. And most horrifying of all, if they want to get from point A to point B, Paris and Nicole have to actually work for it. Or at least pretend to while their supervisors are watching. And apparently the same skills that they use to shop on Madison Avenue do not apply to milking cows, spreading manure, running a switchboard, or making collated copies. And air traffic controllers don't honor American Express platinum cards.

The Simple Life is a great antidote to the workaday blues because it applauds all of us simple-lifers, deep down in the trenches earning our daily bread, for whom life is not really as simple as it might seem. Watching two wayward jet-setters making a mess out of the easiest tasks, and saying all of the things that we wish we could say to our supervisors when they're called on their poor collating skills, is like pure caviar for the put-upon employee in us all. So the next time you're feeling like a serf in the kingdom of life, watch Princesses Paris and Nicole get their meticulously manicured hands dirty, and nibble your virtual revenge on toast points.

■ *Taxi (1978–1983)*
   Stars: Judd Hirsch, Tony Danza, Danny DeVito, Christopher Lloyd,
      Marilu Henner, Andy Kaufman, Jeff Conaway, Carol Kane

A cab company in New York City forms the backdrop for this seventies sitcom about the ups and downs of big-city alienation, and reminds all of us cabbies on the boulevards of life that even if you've got a dead-end job, you're always on the road to somewhere, as long as you have faith in yourself and plenty of gas in your tank.

Taxi takes place in the garage of the Sunshine Cab Company, home to a ragtag group of cabbies all in search of a better life, and more important, a better job. Louie DePalma (Danny DeVito), the cab company's diminutive dictator of a manager, presides from his cage over the lives, loves, and incomes of his employees with a Machiavellian glee, and never misses an opportunity to point out the empty futility in the lives of his drivers. Alex Rieger (Judd Hirsch), the oldest driver in the garage, who's seen it all and come away sadder but wiser, plays the good father to his coworkers, who include: Tony Banta (Tony Danza), a former knockout king who's down for the count; Bobby Wheeler (Jeff Conaway), an aspiring actor with pretty-boy looks and a really bad agent; Elaine Nardo (Marilu Henner), a single gal looking for love in all the wrong places; Jim Ignatowski (Christopher Lloyd), a fading flower child whose brain cells have spent one too many evenings with Timothy Leary, and Latka (Andy Kaufman), the innocent but idiotic immigrant from a country that nobody can pronounce.

As each of these characters struggles to follow the highway of their dreams and break out of the garage forever, and wind up driving straight into the brick wall of reality, Rieger counsels them in the rules of the road and reminds them, along with all of us, that what matters in life is not where you wind up, but keeping your eye on the road and enjoying the ride, because the meter is always running.

TAXI DRIVER WISDOM

Hey, Alex, you know the really great thing about television? If something important happens, anywhere in the world, night or day...
you can always change the channel.
★ Christopher Lloyd as Reverend Jim in *Taxi*

One thing about being a cabbie is that you don't have to worry about being fired from a good job.
★ Judd Hirsch as Alex Rieger in *Taxi*

I wore flowers in my hair and meditated for hours on end. I was finding God all over the place....He kept ditching me.

★ Christopher Lloyd as Reverend Jim in *Taxi*

I'm going to die as I've lived, wearing a green shirt, a catcher's mask, and dancing the cancan.

★ Judd Hirsch as Alex Rieger in *Taxi*

Jason's Minibar—The Grateful Dead

When it's been one of those weeks, and you've been working your fingers to the bone, when Friday finally comes live it up with your crypt-mates with a Grateful Dead on the rocks, to remind yourself that there is life after work. This drink is a modified Long Island Iced Tea, which really packs a wallop, so I want to emphasize that it is made to be *shared* with *all* of the ghouls in your corporate graveyard.

Here's what you'll need:
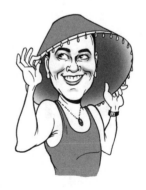
1 part vodka
1 part tequila
1 part rum
1 part gin
1 part triple sec
1½ parts sweet-and-sour mix
1 splash Coca-Cola
Dash grenadine
Lemon slices
Sprig of fresh mint

Here's how you do it:
Place all ingredients except lemon and mint over ice in a shaker, shake vigorously, and pour into an iced-tea glass. Garnish with a lemon slice and a mint sprig.

■ *ER* (1994–)
   Stars: Noah Wyle, Anthony Edwards, Maura Tierney, Goran Visnjic,
      Laura Innes, George Clooney

If you think you had a rough day at the salt mines, spend a few hours in the emergency room at County General, and comfort yourself that as tough as things can get sometimes, at least you don't have to rattle off words like *cardiomyopathy* at breakneck speed while intubating a dispo as a flight-for-life chopper crashes into your intake bay.

Michael Crichton's riveting emergency room drama rolls like a crash cart through the corridors of your workaday doldrums. In each episode a rotating cast of vaguely recognizable and understatedly gorgeous doctors and nurses with really good enunciation skills goes toe-to-toe with disaster, drug addiction, severed limbs, and swollen production budgets. Sometimes they win, sometimes they don't, but the staff at County General always manages to administer some of the best beat-the-job blues ever prescribed, by reminding us that life is fleeting and fragile, and as bad as things can get sometimes, at least you have your health. So the next time your professional vital signs are flagging, let the doctors and nurses of *ER* put the paddles to your chest and zap you back to life, because life is a terrible thing to waste worrying about a job.

MADE-FOR-TV MOVIE MAALOX

The Jacksons: An American Dream (1992)
Stars: Angela Bassett, Lawrence Hilton-Jacobs, Billy Dee Williams, Holly
   Robinson Peete, Margaret Avery, Alex Burrall, Jermaine Jackson II,
   Bumper Robinson, Floyd Roger Myers Jr., Jason Weaver

Before Michael's plastic surgery and court battles, La Toya's *Playboy* spread, and Janet's wardrobe malfunction, the Jacksons were just an average, working-class family nestled quietly in the heart of Gary, Indiana, leading, quiet Gary, Indiana, lives. Yeah, right.

When father Joseph (Lawrence Hilton-Jacobs) discovers that his sons can really sing, the Jacksons' long day's journey into night begins. From gigging at local venues to low-budget tours through the backwater bars of middle America, the Jacksons hump it Partridge-style, selling their sound, until Motown comes a-callin' and launches The Jackson 5 into pop culture history and infamy.

Although this miniseries doesn't dive enough into the abuse, the scandals, and the pressure from big bad Joe to classify this movie as true camp (and this is a real shame), there is enough of an eyeful here to make you realize that maybe becoming a pop star like you always dreamed you'd be isn't such a sweet deal after all. This movie is a great reminder that no matter how glamorous somebody else's job may seem on the surface, you always have to sing for your supper.

■ *The Apprentice (2004–)*

Misery loves company, so if you've had a rough day at the office, sometimes it can be comforting to watch somebody else make a worse mess of things than you ever could, and hear those magic words "You're fired" without having to look for a new career direction in the morning.

Donald Trump's reality show brings together sixteen contestants from all walks of life, from Harvard MBA grads to street vendors, and puts them into a corporate setting to see who is the baddest ass in the boardroom, we mean besides Donald Trump and his platinum enforcer Carolyn (now, *that's* a celebrity smack-down we'd like to see).

The carrot they dangle in front of these mismatched and often disgruntled would-be extreme execs is the promise of a job in the Trump organization, at a salary of a quarter of a million dollars a year. Each week contestants are broken up into two teams, given a task, like selling Trump water, inventing and marketing a new flavor of ice cream, or running a pedicab. While the teams struggle to sink or swim in the white water of big-city business, we get to sit back, crack open a cold one, and watch them sputter and stall on the road to success.

Not only is *The Apprentice* a great cure for a bad day at the office, but we really do learn a lot about doing business in the process. *The Apprentice* teaches us that business really isn't just business, that a multibillion-dollar deal requires many of the same skills as selling a glass of lemonade, that the Omarosas of the world do ultimately get what's coming to them, and that in the end, the best team still wins.

TRUMPISMS

Experience taught me a few things. One is to listen to your gut, no matter how good something sounds on paper. The second is that you're generally better off sticking with what you know. And the third is that sometimes your best investments are the ones you don't make.

I like thinking big. If you're going to be thinking anything, you might as well think big.

I try to learn from the past, but I plan for the future by focusing exclusively on the present. That's where the fun is.

I wasn't satisfied just to earn a good living. I was looking to make a statement.

Money was never a big motivation for me, except as a way to keep score. The real excitement is playing the game.

Part of being a winner is knowing when enough is enough. Sometimes you have to give up the fight and walk away, and move on to something that's more productive.

What separates the winners from the losers is how a person reacts to each new twist of fate.

I have a bad haircut!

★ all quotes from Donald Trump in *The Apprentice*

■ *The Office (2001–2003)*
  Stars: Ricky Gervais, Martin Freeman, Mackenzie Crook, Lucy Davis,
    Patrick Baladi

If you're in the mood to roast your boss and serve him up for supper, have a triple help-ing of this British "mockumentary" about a floundering and obscure paper company in the wasteland of the English Midlands, and let off some of your pent-up steam with laughter instead of larceny.

David Brent (Ricky Gervais) presides over an office full of disgruntled underlings all scrambling to hold on to their dead-end jobs in a dead-end economy in a dead-end town in a dead-end industry. This means, of course, that they have to humor their dead-end boss, who thinks he is the best thing since sliced cheese…emphasis on the word *cheese*. As the handheld camera follows the leader, documentary style, through the ins and outs of his workday, David, who genuinely believes that he is a midlevel celebrity instead of a midlevel tyrant, struts and frets his hour upon his petty stage. His staff members, including dishy blonde receptionist Dawn (Lucy Davis), office rebel Tim Canterbury (Martin Freeman), and office yes-man Garth (Mackenzie Crook), hold their noses and try their best not to laugh in Dave's moon face. So the next time you're feeling the boot of managerial oppres-sion, spend a few hours in Slough with the employees of *The Office* and engage in a little of nature's best medicine, at the boss's expense.

DAVID'S DELUSIONS OF GRANDEUR

Those of you who think you know everything are annoying to those of us
who do.

When confronted by a difficult problem, you can solve it more easily by
reducing it to the question "How would the Lone Ranger handle this?"

Well, there's good news and bad news. The bad news is that Neil will be taking over both branches, and some of you will lose your jobs. On a more positive note, the good news is, I've been promoted, so...every cloud. You're still thinking about the bad news, aren't you?

And if it's ideas for TV shows, game shows, or whatever you want, I'm your man. I'm already exploring the entertainment avenue with my management training, but I'd like to do that on a global scale really.

What is the single most important thing for a company? Is it the building? Is it the stock? Is it the turnover? It's the people, investment in people. My proudest moment here wasn't when I increased profits by 17 percent or cut expenditure without losing a single member of staff. No. It was a young Greek guy, first job in the country, hardly spoke a word of English, but he came to me and he went, "Mr. Brent, will you be the godfather to my child?" Didn't happen in the end. We had to let him go, he was rubbish.

★ all quotes from Ricky Gervais as David Brent in *The Office*

SISTERS ARE DOIN' IT FOR THEMSELVES

In the seventies, a raft of shows appeared on the network airwaves featuring women who left their traditional roles as moms and wives and hit the road in search of a better job and a better future. So the next time you're feeling like you missed the exit ramp that leads to the highway of professional happiness, hit the road with these female TV mavericks, and discover along with them that you really can change your life just by changing your career.

One Day at a Time (1975–1984)
Stars: Bonnie Franklin, Pat Harrington Jr., Valerie Bertinelli, Mackenzie Phillips

After seventeen years of marriage, perky redhead Ann Romano (Bonnie Franklin) finds herself divorced, and moves to Indianapolis with her daughters,

Barbara (Valerie Bertinelli) and Julie (Mackenzie Phillips during the Studio 54 years, if you catch our drift), and begins to build a new career, a new family, and a new life.

Ann and her typical teen daughters are immediately adopted by their building's super, Schneider (Pat Harrington), who fixes pipes about as well as he fixes family problems, but whose heart is always in the right place. Ann, like many women at the time this series ran, must reenter the job market for the first time since her marriage, but moves rapidly up the corporate ladder from secretary, to ad exec, to the owner of her own agency, and grows out of the seventies into a successful and independent career woman of the eighties. This all proves that there really is life after divorce and you can live your life on your own terms as long as you are willing to let go of your preconceptions, build family where you find it, and bank on your talents.

Alice (1976–1985)
Stars: Linda Lavin, Philip McKeon, Vic Tayback, Beth Howland,
Polly Holiday

When her husband dies unexpectedly, leaving her with a teenage son, Tommy, and no future prospects, Alice (Linda Lavin) heads for Hollywood to pursue her dream of becoming a singer. Unfortunately, her beat-up Buick has other ideas, and when she breaks down in Phoenix, Alice takes a job at Mel's Diner to earn the money to repair her car.

Mel (Vic Tayback), the owner of the diner, is a tough-as-nails fry cook who's pure mashed potatoes underneath. And Alice's greasy spoon sisters include Flo "kiss my grits" Castleberry (Polly Holiday), who has a red bouffant so high she has to register it with the FAA, and a sharp tongue capable of cutting anybody down to size, who teaches Alice how to reenter the dating world and the working life.

Soon, what started out as a stopgap measure on the road to bigger dreams come true turns into the new job, home, and family that Alice would never have planned on, and she puts down roots in her new short-order home, where love, comfort, down-to-earth wisdom, and good humor are always on the menu.

▪ *Six Feet Under (2001–)*
  Stars: *Michael C. Hall, Peter Krause, Frances Conroy, Lauren Ambrose,*
    Rachel Griffiths, Freddy Rodriguez, Matthew St. Patrick

If you're feeling buried up to your eyeballs in your office plots, spend some time with the Fishers, who have made a career out of facing death and endure an infinity of existential dilemmas.

Mother Ruth (Frances Conroy) is the new head of the household in a family-run funeral home in Pasadena that sells comfort to the bereaved and final rest to the dearly departed. When Ruth suddenly finds herself widowed, she must construct a brand-new life in this house of death. In fact, all of the characters in creator Alan Ball's (*American Beauty*) macabre family dramedy are searching, each in his or her own way, to be reborn from the ashes of a dysfunctional past and to keep their personal problems from interfering with the implacable calm and serenity they must present to their customers.

Nate (Peter Krause), the golden boy who got away, is forced to grow up and shoulder the weight of the family business and bury the teenager within, who just wants to shrug the whole thing off and go get laid. David (Michael C. Hall), the younger Fisher son, is struggling with his sexual identity while living in his big brother's shadow. And then there's Claire (Lauren Ambrose), the rebellious teenage daughter who is going through the anti-everything phase.

Yet despite the death that surrounds the Fishers on the job and off, they are all brimming with life. Perhaps it's because being on a first-name basis with death puts us on more intimate terms with its alternative. The Fisher family's weekly funeral reminds all of us working stiffs that when all is said and done, the petty concerns of our day-to-day lives come to a heap of ashes, and the only thing that really matters in life is love.

QUOTES FROM THE CRYPT

Look, I have to go identify our dead father's body. I'm sorry you're having a bad drug experience, but deal with it.

★ Peter Krause as Nate in *Six Feet Under*

Well, well. The prodigal returns. This is what you've been running away from your whole life, buddy boy. Scared the crap out of you when you were growing up, didn't it? And you thought you'd escape, well, guess what, nobody escapes.

★ Richard Jenkins as Nate Sr. in *Six Feet Under*

I know stealing a foot is weird. But, hello, living in a house where a foot is available to be stolen is weird.

★ Lauren Ambrose as Claire in *Six Feet Under*

If we live our lives the right way, then everything we do can become a work of art.

★ Lauren Ambrose as Claire in *Six Feet Under*

■ *Family Plots (2004)*

Reality TV meets *Six Feet Under* in this episodic look at the inner workings of a family-run mortuary in a San Diego suburb. The star of this funeral home is Shana Bernardo, the head embalmer, who has no problem preserving bodies but is too empathetic and emotional to comfort grieving families, even though she is the head consoler in her own. She is assisted by her sisters Melissa and Emily, her ex-boxer father Chuck, a softhearted lug of a man who loves and irritates his daughters with equal measure, and Rick, the owner of the funeral home, who has an on-again, off-again romance with Melissa. Yet despite the death, and the grief, and the gross stuff that goes on behind the closed doors of a mortuary, the Bernardos are happy in their work because they know that what they're doing makes a big difference in the lives of people in distress. *Family Plots* reminds us that death is not nearly as scary as working in a family-run business, but also reassures us that working together creates an unshakable bond, and the family that works together, stays together.

Bev's TV Tray: Sweet Hereafter Bread

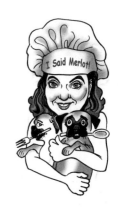

Because a piece of this delicious bread tastes like a little slice of heaven, just when you need it most.

Here's what you'll need:
1/2 cup butter or margarine, softened
1 cup sugar
2 eggs
1 cup mashed bananas
3 tablespoons whole-berry cranberry sauce
2 cups sifted flour
1 1/4 teaspoons baking powder
1 teaspoon baking soda
1/2 teaspoon salt
1 cup white chocolate chips
1 cup chopped walnuts

Here's how you do it:
In a large bowl cream butter and sugar thoroughly. Add eggs one at a time and beat well. Stir in mashed bananas and cranberries. Combine flour, baking powder, baking soda, and salt, and add to the batter. Fold in white chocolate chips and nuts and pour into a greased baking pan. Bake at 350 degrees for 55 to 60 minutes. Cool thoroughly before slicing. This bread tastes like a little bit of deliverance in a pan.

CHAPTER 5

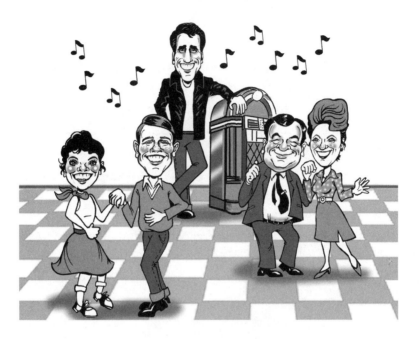

Teen Spirit TV

ADOLESCENCE ISN'T JUST AN age, it's a state of mind, and it doesn't come around only once in life. The same is true in television land, where teendom seems to crop up on every spin of the dial. Perhaps it's because we all long to go home again and relive a little of our youthful innocence, only in a better zip code. Maybe it's also because we all have an inner teenager who breaks out like a pimple on prom night every time we try out a new skill or stretch forward into new territory. Growth always involves a little awkwardness and can leave us feeling a little gangly, a little foolish, and Teen Spirit TV helps remind us that we're not alone and we will survive. So if you're a teenager of any age, let these timeless heroes and heroines reassure you that there is no gain without a little pain, and that if you made it through adolescence, you can make it through anything.

▪ *The O.C. (2003–)*
  Stars: Peter Gallagher, Benjamin McKenzie, Kelly Rowan, Adam Brody,
    Mischa Barton, Rachel Bilson

TV's favorite adolescent smolderer, Ryan Atwood (Benjamin McKenzie), is a teen hero with a cynical twist, who, like the Fresh Prince before him, introduces a touch of the mean streets into the affluent and carefree zip codes of Southern California. Ryan grows up in unfashionable Chino with a felonious brother, an alcoholic mother, and few, if any, prospects for the future. When Ryan is picked up by the police for helping his brother steal a car, he's rescued from ignominy and certain self-destruction by his public defender, Sandy Cohen (Peter Gallagher), a paternal figure for a retro-eighties America, now that fathers once again always know best. Accompanied by his new brother, Seth (Adam Brody), a geek in the land of cool and hence, like Ryan, a stranger in a strange land, and his snappy girlfriend, Marissa (Mischa Barton), Ryan must learn along with the rest of us that while money can't buy you love, it definitely makes it easier to come of age. But we and all of the residents of sunny Orange County also learn that wealth and privilege alone mean nothing if you grow up without the fertile soil of a loving and supportive community of family and friends, who will be there as soon as you reach out for them.

So, if you've been feeling like a fish out of water and you're finding it a little difficult to breathe, let the kids and parents of *The O.C.* remind you that no matter where the current takes you in life, you'll always stay afloat as long as you hold fast to the rudder and know when to call for all hands on deck.

LOVE STINKS

Drinking, crying, cops, well it must be Christmas.
  ★ Benjamin McKenzie as Ryan Atwood in *The O.C.*

Never underestimate a parent's ability to mortify his child.
  ★ Peter Gallagher as Sandy Cohen in *The O.C.*

Your love triangle is more like a love rhombus.
★ Adam Brody as Seth Cohen in *The O.C.*

God, he loves you. He got into a fight and burned down a house over you. That's hot.
★ Rachel Bilson as Summer Roberts in *The O.C.*

I knew it was only a matter of time before you started bringing home felons.
★ Kelly Rowan as Kirsten Cohen in *The O.C.*

■ *Made (2003)*

High school teens reach for dreams they could never normally accomplish—with a little help from MTV. An average-looking girl runs for homecoming queen . . . and takes the crown; a high school jock learns how to ballet-dance to win the girl of his dreams; and a southern belle with a little baby fat learns how to go the distance on an extreme biking course to catch the attention of the boy next door. This may sound like a setup for a real disaster—and while it's true that some of these teens don't necessarily make their dreams come true in quite the ways they'd hoped, many do. They all, however, gain an invaluable life lesson about the value of stretching beyond their comfort zones, and becoming more than they thought they could be, whether or not the guy or girl of their dreams happens to notice. This show also takes direct aim at the classism of high school that keeps some kids well to the left of center stage who really shine once the spotlight is turned on them.

If you've been feeling like you're out with the in crowd in the high school of life, and like no matter how hard you rally you're never going to make the cheer squad, let the kids of *Made* remind you that you are only as popular as you think you are, and that the pom-poms go to the students of life who believe in themselves.

▪ *Sweet Sixteen (2005–)*

MTV cameras follow fifteen-year-olds from all walks of life as they prepare for and ultimately attend the sweet sixteen party of their dreams. And on a show with a tag line that reads "Because sometimes sixteen isn't so sweet," we're pretty much prepared right from the get-go for some world-class party pique. And we get it in spades. Rather like a junior version of *Bridezilla*, this show follows kids who will stop at nothing to make their sweet-sixteen fantasies come true. And, as we discover, sixteen-year-olds have some pretty adult party fantasies, with some very adult party budgets. From two best friends who have obviously taken a few tips from Paris and Nicole—whose party hair, clothes, and shoe budgets alone must exceed the national debt of a small country—to a girl who wants a simple gathering in defiance of her mom's four-star Mardi Gras dreams, to a New York City son of a professional party planner who hires girls to attend his bash and even buys them a party wardrobe, these kids battle against bossy or overly indulgent parents, jealous siblings, and out-of-control party guests to make their sweet-sixteen visions a reality. And many of them learn, along with their parents who are footing the bill, to be careful what you wish for because you just might get it.

If you're feeling like a wallflower in the coming-out party of life, let these super sweet sixteens remind you that what makes a good sweet-sixteen party is having your friends and family gather around you to wish you well as you enter a new phase of independence, and not the label on your gown, the length of your limo, or the size of your bottom line.

▪ *Beverly Hills 90210 (1990–2000)*
  Stars: Shannen Doherty, Jason Priestley, Jennie Garth, Ian Ziering,
    Gabrielle Carteris, Luke Perry, Brian Austin Green, Tori Spelling

If you're longing for a simpler, younger time when comfort and friendship were as close and effortless as the next lunch period, then come on down to the Peach Pit and hang out with the kids of Beverly Hills High School, who remind us that as long as Aaron Spelling and Darren Star are alive and well in TV-land, you really can go home again, at least for a few hours.

This groundbreaking series, which in many ways set the stage for *Friends* and won the hearts of America for a decade, revolves around the lives and loves of a group of upper-middle-class and upper-class, not to mention exceedingly well-scrubbed and untypical, teenagers, who live in one of the most desirable zip codes in the world. The kids of *Beverly Hills 90210*—Brenda (Shannen Doherty), Brandon (Jason Priestley), Kelly (Jennie Garth), Andrea (Gabrielle Carteris), Steve (Ian Ziering), Dylan (Luke Perry), Donna (Tori Spelling), and David (Brian Austin Green)—seem to have completely bypassed the awkwardness of adolescence. Nobody even gets a pimple and everybody's teeth are perfectly straight. Yet they do wrestle with their share of Beverly Hills TV dilemmas. They fall in love, they fall out of love, they plan parties, and they struggle with peer pressure, teen alcoholism, even apartheid.

Yet no matter what this group of Beverly Hills teens wrestles with over a whole decade, they never encounter anything—not anti-Semitism or alcoholism or AIDS, or apparently even the effects of aging—that can't be cured with a low-fat latte down at the Peach Pit, a fireside chat with Mom and Pop Walsh, and a little help from their friends.

WORDS TO LIVE BY

Andrea, this is California. Blondes are like the state flower or something.
★ Ian Ziering as Steve in *Beverly Hills 90210*

So I was blitz shopping Melrose yesterday, and I see Jockey for her, Calvin Klein for her, BVD for her. Now, I don't get it, I mean, I don't see them making Maidenform for him.
★ Tori Spelling as Donna in *Beverly Hills 90210*

Aren't you supposed to toss the car when the oil's dirty?
★ Ian Ziering as Steve in *Beverly Hills 90210*

You'll have to forgive Donna, Mr. Canner. You see, she thinks it's a
tragedy to leave home without her gold card.
★ Jennie Garth as Kelly in *Beverly Hills 90210*

All is fair in love and volleyball.
★ Luke Perry as Dylan in *Beverly Hills 90210*

▪ *My So-Called Life* (1994–1995)
   Stars: Claire Danes, Bess Armstrong, Wilson Cruz, A. J. Langer,
      Jared Leto

Angela Chase (Claire Danes) is the voice of teen angst in this short-lived but critically celebrated series, which gives us a terrifying and all-too-familiar look back into the both fragile and Herculean heart of a teenage girl. And because she is a teenage girl, Angela struggles with the usual menu of parent issues, complexion problems (there's even an episode called "The Zit"), peer pressure, and, of course, *boys*. Angela's teenage crush is on bad boy Jordan Catalano (Jared Leto), who can't put more than three words together to form a sentence and never expresses his feelings, but who looks *fabulous* when he pouts, particularly when he is wearing jeans and a skimpy T-shirt. Together with her best friends, Rayanne (A. J. Langer), who is voted the biggest potential slut in high school, and Ricky (Wilson Cruz), who is struggling to come out of the closet, Angela rides the tide of her development and fights to keep her head above water as the waves of her childhood crash onto the shore and deposit her, somewhat dazed, on the beach of young adulthood. So if you're feeling like a ship without a home port in a sea of the unknown, let *My So-Called Life* remind you that even though the seas may get a little rough sometimes, you'll always find your way to a sandy shore, as long as you keep your hands on the wheel and trust your ability to sail your own ship.

ANGELA'S ASHES

Sometimes it seems like we're all living in some kind of prison.
And the crime is how much we hate ourselves.

The worst feeling is suddenly realizing that you don't measure up. And
that, in the past, when you thought you did, you were a fool.

I'm in love. His name is Jordan Catalano. He was left back, twice. He's
always closing his eyes like it hurts to look at things.

Seeing a teacher's actual lunch is, like, so depressing. Not to
mention her bra strap.

Lately, I can't even look at my mother without wanting
to stab her repeatedly.

School is a battlefield for your heart. So when Rayanne Graff told me my
hair was holding me back, I had to listen. 'Cause she wasn't just talking
about my hair. She was talking about my life.

★ all quotes from Claire Danes as Angela in My So-Called Life

▪ *Happy Days (1974–1984)*
Stars: Ron Howard, Henry Winkler, Tom Bosley, Marion Ross, Erin
Moran, Anson Williams, Don Most

America's favorite everyteen, Ron Howard, stars as Richie Cunningham, a teenager in Wisconsin in the fifties who struggles to overcome his insecurities, his unreliable complexion, and the most alarming collection of plaid button-downs ever assembled in order to find his thrill on Blueberry Hill. Assisting him in his quest for manhood are his parents, Marion (Marion Ross) and Howard (Tom Bosley), who were a new brand of TV parents who actually had a sense of humor about themselves, and his sister, Joannie (Erin Moran), who bounces around in a poodle skirt until she finally gets her own teen spin-off. And Richie has his friends Potsy (Anson Williams), the lovable lug, and Ralph Malph (Don Most), the geek on the block who makes all his friends look better by comparison. And then there's the iconic Arthur Fonzarelli (Henry Winkler), who manages to overcome monosyllabic dialogue, fifth billing, and even middle age to become one of America's favorite visions of teenage cool, and who teaches Richie everything his father can't about how to get the girl.

So if you're feeling overwhelmed by the complexities of coming of age in a new millennium and are longing for the good old days that never were, rock around the clock with Richie Cunningham and the *Happy Days* gang, for whom growing up is as easy as sipping cider through a straw.

Jason's Minibar—The Cherry Float

When you're strolling down memory lane, make a pit stop at the place when there was nothing that couldn't be cured with carbonation, two scoops of ice cream, and a cherry on top.

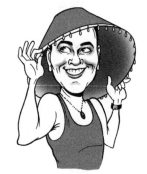

Here's what you'll need:
> *2 scoops vanilla ice cream*
> *Maraschino cherries (and the juice)*
> *Bottle of Coca-Cola*
> *Whipped cream*
> *Frosted mug*

Here's how you do it:
> *Place the vanilla ice cream and a splash of cherry juice into your mug and pour in some ice-cold Coca-Cola. Garnish with whipped cream and a cherry and eat yourself up, up, and away to a place where you can't get into any trouble and chocolate never makes you break out.*

GEEK TV

Go ahead, nobody's watching. Pull the blinds, dim the lights, pour a few thousand empty calories in a bowl, and indulge your inner nerd with some good old-fashioned Geek TV featuring classic unhipsters who remind us that cool is measured by the quality of your character, not the brand of your shoes.

Freaks and Geeks (1999–2000)
*Stars: Linda Cardellini, John Francis Daley, James Franco, Samm
  Levine, Seth Rogen, Jason Segel, Martin Starr, Becky Ann
  Baker, Joe Flaherty, Busy Phillips*

Freaks and Geeks is an uncomfortably accurate reminiscence about what high school was really like for the rest of us, puts us all back in that high-school auditorium of yesteryear, and lets us watch the struggles of adolescence without Aaron Spelling and Darren Star's rose-colored lenses. This is a teen show about the kids outside of the high-school limelight—the ones who are hanging out under the bleachers and getting a different kind of education: the kind you get when you are trapped on the underside and looking up at life. The heroes of *Freaks and Geeks* are the dweebs who aren't on the cheer squad or the football team or even the yearbook committee, but rather spend their wonder years on the outskirts of high-school society, struggling to come of age in a world that doesn't appreciate them. This unusual and intelligent teen soap opera focuses on the Weir teenagers, who both, somewhat reluctantly, attend McKinley High School. Lindsay (Linda Cardellini) is a sixteen-year-old overachieving mathlete who finally hits breaking point when her grandmother dies. To express her teen angst, she eschews her inner geeky good girl and starts hanging out under the bleachers with bad boy Daniel (James Franco) in a green flak jacket, while listening to Led Zeppelin at full volume and discussing the ultimate futility of all human endeavors. Sound familiar? Lindsay's younger brother Sam (John Francis Daley), literally a 98-pound weakling who ought to be wearing a sign that says KICK SAND AT ME, struggles to stay alive in a jungle of jocks with the help of his fellow inhabitants of dorkville, Neal (Samm Levine) and Bill (Martin Starr). This startlingly accurate series, which was sadly canceled in its infancy, much to the dismay of its many cult followers, gives us all a startling and hilarious firsthand look into the hidden life of geeks, and gives us all a pretty good idea why it's usually the nerds in high school who succeed in life—because when you're used to coming second in life, you just learn to try harder.

GEEK WISDOM

We're all unhappy. That's the thing about life.
★ Linda Cardellini as Lindsay Weir in *Freaks and Geeks*

I'm Jewish. That's no cakewalk either. Last year, I was elected school treasurer. I didn't even run!
★ Samm Levine as Neal Schweiber in *Freaks and Geeks*

Hey, I believe in god, man. I've seen him, I've felt his power! He plays drums for Led Zeppelin and his name is John Bonham, baby!
★ Jason Segel as Nick Andopolis in *Freaks and Geeks*

Are you calling me irrational? Because I'll tear your head off, Daniel. I'll tear it off and I'll throw it over that fence.
★ Busy Phillips as Kim Kelly in *Freaks and Geeks*

Strangers with Candy *(1999–2000 and 2005)*
Stars: Amy Sedaris, Stephen Colbert, Paul Dinello

Amy Sedaris stars as Jerri Blank, a forty-six-year-old supergeek, a self-proclaimed "user, boozer, and loser," who cleans up her act and picks up where she left off thirty-two years ago—as a dork in high school. Set against an ideal suburban backdrop, Jerri struggles to learn important teenage lessons she got wrong the first time around—like you can't buy love from the popular girls with homemade hallucinogens, and that for some people, it's better to be boozed up all the time, because they're just too plain mean to be sober.

As Jerri staggers and stumbles through this after-school-special neverland, assaulting every golden rule in the book, she provides us with a hilarious and strangely comforting reassurance that as dweebie as we might all feel at times, there is always Jerri, standing her ground out there on the borderlines of bad taste and shooting us the moon. This series—which was created by and stars Amy Sedaris, Stephen Colbert, and Paul Dinello, three well-seasoned Second City vets—looks right in the face of the darkest and most disturbing images of youthful innocence lost and geekdom found, and laughs right out loud.

JERRI'S LEFT JABS

If you're gonna reach for a star, reach for the lowest one you can.

I cried when I had no shoes. Then I saw a man who had no feet. And then I laughed really hard.

I'm not adopted and I'm not an Indian. It's just a coincidence that I have a love of gambling and booze and a knack for catching syphilis.

Orlando, you can't be a pilgrim. The pilgrims had snowy white skin to match their pure Christian souls. They didn't sacrifice coconuts to their monkey gods.

I'm guessing this is a dream. Only difference is you're not naked and tied to a radiator.

Florida. Beautiful weather—harsh penal system.
★ all quotes from Amy Sedaris as Jerri Blank in *Strangers with Candy*

The Christopher Lowell Show (1999–)

Christopher Lowell, the king geek of decorating, is to interior design what Charo is to music, and with both, you need a translator to understand what the hell is going on.

With his touch screen, glue gun, and whole cast of visiting vendors, Christopher Lowell packed up his career building TV sets and moved to his own show, where he teaches us that even nerds can have a home that looks like a stage set or a department store window.

Giving us part permission and part encouragement to be creative, Mr. Lowell teaches us in each show how to break out of our white-wall thinking and emerge into a merchandised, colorful world of better living and a better sense of our interior designer self.

We can't help but love Christopher's drive and his ability to laugh at himself (we are laughing *with* him, right?), but I can't help but be disturbed and in awe of each episode's opening segment. It's like we start out in a dark basement of a late-night drag show (starring you-know-who as a mermaid, a little geek boy, an old woman, and even Ms. Martha Stewart herself), and then suddenly find ourselves just as suddenly transported into our grandmother's living room filled with home and craft projects. And doilies. This is geek chic at its campiest.

So when you're looking for a show that is going to make you feel a little bit better about your own little corner of the world, tune in for some of Christopher's decorating, crafting, draping, building, buying, arranging, party-planning color courage and remember, YOU CAN DO IT!

Pee-Wee's Playhouse (1986–1990)
*Stars: Paul Reubens, John Paragon, Gregory Harrison,
Phil Hartman*

Pee-Wee's Playhouse was originally intended to be a children's show, and admittedly it was a great way for kids to start their day because it encouragedself-expression and helped kids realize that even the dorky dude in the funny suit with the weird laugh and the bow tie could be fun to hang around with if you gave him a chance. But Pee-Wee also resonated for adults hungry for a little innocent Romper Room recreation and the permission to be the dorks that we are, if only for a few moments, in the privacy of our darkened home theater. At Pee-Wee's, kooky is cool, dweebie is divine, and anything is acceptable as long as it feels good and doesn't hurt anybody else. Along with Pee-Wee's guests, we are reminded to "scream real loud" when each day's secret word is said and are encouraged to be as wacky and wild and dorky as possible. This show stretches the limits of our possibilities and reminds all of us who are a little afraid to shout out that when you find the courage to express yourself, good things can and will happen, even if you look kinda goofy while you're doing it.

■ *Party of Five* (1994–2000)
  Stars: Matthew Fox, Scott Wolf, Neve Campbell, Lacey Chabert,
  Jennifer Love Hewitt

When their parents are killed by a drunk driver, five kids, who range in age from baby-hood to twentysomething, must raise each other in an affluent California suburb, ever mindful that if they don't do a good job of it, they may lose the privilege of growing up to-gether. Now, this is a lot for any teenager to handle, let alone two teenage siblings who must both spend at least two and a half hours in the gym every day, not to mention the mainte-nance that must go into those highlights. On, yeah, and they have to go to class.

At the head of the Salinger household is Charlie (Matthew Fox), a ruggedly handsome barely postadolescent surrogate father who is like a Ward Cleaver in training, only single, and with better abs (see note above re: two and a half hours daily in the gym). Next in line is sister Julia (Neve Campbell's debut), who is beautiful in an Ivory Soap sense, and who you just know is going to turn out to be the ideal American soccer mom one day, no mat-ter how many times she gets pregnant out of wedlock beforehand. Next in line is Bailey (Scott Wolf), the teenage stud who courts a dangerous relationship with liquid courage, but who we just know is a nice all-American boy underneath all that bourbon and bad behav-ior. And we never really doubt that his super sweet and supportive girlfriend (Jennifer Love

Hewitt) will one day help him turn his life around. And then there's tweenager Claudia (Lacey Chabert), who struggles against these three resident scenery-chewers for her share of screen time. Think Jan Brady, only with more interesting hair and no glasses. Oh, and there's a baby in there somewhere, too, whom Julia has to take care of every once in a while, between her yoga class and her deep facial. Together this family must not only take over adult roles beyond their level of development, but cope at the same time with the familiar pangs of adolescence.

Party of Five quickly developed a devoted audience, which was so passionate that they flooded the network with letters when the series was canceled, forcing TV executives to change their mind and pick up the show for another season. We're not sure if *Party of Five* inspired such enthusiastic viewer support because it brought our worst nightmares to life, or because it gave us a forbidden glimpse of our wildest teenage dreams come true. A world without parents is both a thrilling and a terrifying notion when you are fourteen. Regardless, *Party of Five* reminds us of the strength and resilience of the bond that exists between siblings, and brings us back to an age and a place when the only thing that stood between us and chaos was the love and stability of our sisters and brothers.

■ *Dawson's Creek* (1998–2003)
  Stars: *James Van Der Beek, Katie Holmes, Joshua Jackson, Michelle
  Williams, Kerr Smith*

Welcome to the *Melrose Place* of teendom, where for the kids of *Dawson's Creek* growing up is made even harder by the limitations of their small town.

Dawson (James Van Der Beek) and Joey (Katie Holmes) are lifelong best friends whose relationship suddenly changes when their hormones begin to flow. These two friends and lovers struggle to define their feelings for each other while their star-crossed friend Pacey (Joshua Jackson) struggles to find his place in the whole mix.

The most interesting thing about this small-town teen soap opera is that the adults act more like teenagers than the kids. The parents in *Dawson's Creek* are forever fouling things up, leaving it to their freakishly perceptive and emotionally mobile kids to clean up the mess.

So when all of the adults in your life start acting like unruly kids, spend a few hours in Capeside, and let the teens of *Dawson's Creek* teach you how to turn the tables.

JOEY'S JUJUBES

Hang on, Dawson, it's gonna be a bumpy life.

I just think our emerging hormones are destined to alter our relationship...
and I'm trying to limit the fallout.

I thought this was what I wanted—for you to see me as beautiful, for you to look at me the way you look at Jen. But the truth is I don't want that, I don't want that at all. I want you to look at me and see the person you've always known and realize that what we have is so much more important than just some passing physical attraction, 'cause you know what, Dawson? It's just lipstick and it's just hair spray. You've had a lifetime to process your feelings for me, and I can't spend the rest of mine hoping you might throw a general glance in my direction between your tortured teen romances with whatever Jen Lindley rolls into your life next—I can't do it.

★ all quotes from Katie Holmes as Joey in *Dawson's Creek*

TEEN ANGST TV

Because sometimes, all of us terrible teens need to get our ya-ya's out.

Jackass (2000–2001)

Jackass is the *Candid Camera* of the angry teen within. With these stuntmen and extreme sports nuts, going too far isn't in their vocabulary. Some of the stunts are hysterical, while others are masochistic and go for the ouch factor, while still others wind up just this side of homoerotic. And why are these guys always naked? These terrible inner teens snort earthworms, shop in G-strings, and wrestle a real bear while dressed like one, just because they can. And for some reason, it's really cathartic. So when you're feeling the need to let go of some of that repressed rage or indulge your inner idiot, spend some time with these jackasses rather than making one out of yourself.

JACKASS JEWELS

Dude, you're the crappiest human bowling ball I ever saw in my whole life.
★ Johnny Knoxville on *Jackass*

I'm sick of the whole pooping thing…I'm gonna go get my butt cheeks pierced together.
★ Steve-O on *Jackass*

I'm Bam Margera, and I feel like kicking my dad's ass all day today!
★ Bam Margera on *Jackass*

I gotta be horrible at everything; otherwise it just wouldn't be me.
★ Ryan Dunn on *Jackass*

South Park (1997–)
Stars: Trey Parker, Matt Stone, Mary Kay Bergman, Jesse Howell, Isaac Hayes, Francesca Clifford, Eliza Schneider

Welcome to the small dysfunctional town of South Park, Colorado, the home of Kenny, Stan, Cartman, and Kyle, the psycho pals who form the nucleus of an animated grammar-school world that plays a lot like a perverse *Peanuts*.

When these trash-talking fourth-graders aren't in school, they are usually hanging out on the wrong side of town involved with UFOs, erupting volcanoes, Big Gay Al, and scatological similes of every conceivable shape and size.

South Park is a great rage reliever, as it reminds us that we shouldn't be too hard on ourselves or each other, because the surreality of small-town life could turn just about anybody into an animated, anally fixated Kenny killer…even good old Charlie Brown himself. So when you're feeling like going postal, tune in to *South Park* and let Kenny and the kids give voice to your dark side, and keep the Anytown USA teen angst on the screen, where it belongs.

THE STRAIGHT POOP

How come everything today has involved things either coming in or going out of my ass?
★ Trey Parker as Cartman in *South Park*

Well, you know. You'll just be sitting there, minding your own business, and they'll come marching in, and crawl up your leg, and start biting the inside of your ass, and you'll be all like "Hey. Get out of my ass, you stupid rainbows." I'm talking about rainbows. I hate those friggin' things.
★ Trey Parker as Cartman in *South Park*

Genetic engineering is a way to fix God's horrible mistakes, like German people.
★ Trey Parker as Mr. Garrison in *South Park*

Look, kid, we just thought it was a bad movie. Tell us how we can get in touch with Mel Gibson so we can get our money back.
★ Trey Parker as Stan in *South Park*

Stan, you need to lay off the cough syrup, all right, seriously. I'm worried about you, man.
★ Trey Parker as Cartman in *South Park*

And then I always get woken up to the sound of my own screams. Do you think I'm unhappy?
★ Matt Stone as Leopold Butters Stotch in *South Park*

TEEN MARVELS

These Marvel Comics heroes, picked up off the pages of comic books and set to life on TV, have become icons for generations of teenagers who were hungry for a role model who wasn't afraid of his inner adolescent. These Marvel superheroes understand the fear and insecurity of adolescence, they know what it means to feel like a freak, and yet they embrace their differences, put their fear into gear, and find the courage to stand up for what they believe in and to be their own person.

Spider-Man *(1967–1970)*
Star: Paul Soles

Young Peter Parker (Paul Soles) is bitten by an irradiated spider in this animated series, and wakes up a web-slinging wonder with the ability to scale walls, knit webs internally, and fly through the air with the greatest of ease. Struggling to understand his new powers, but spurred on by the robbery of his surrogate parents' home, Spider-Man decides to swing with the web of fate and vows to use his superpowers to fight criminals, birdbrains, feathered finks, and grapefruit-heads wherever he finds them. Spider-Man, who had a Clint Eastwood–like dialogue track and was the only superhero in history who never wore a cape, reassures the insecure teenager in us all that while we may feel like an insect, we really can be heroes, if just for one day.

SPIDEY'S WEBS

Hey, what's that? Holy flying catfish! Another superhero . . . or I'm a hallucinating webhead! Great golly-wockles! He can really fly! I wonder who he is. I don't recognize the costume at all. Hey you! What's the big idea of butting in on my turf!

Winging from building to building! Running around in a hot costume!
Sometimes, I wonder why.

Well, here goes. I hope I get the job. Of course, with my spider-power, I
could get all the money I'd ever need, but that wouldn't
be honest. I'm a crime-fighter now.

Yes, Uncle Ben is dead, and in a sense it was really I who killed him.
Because I didn't realize in time that with great power there must also
always be great responsibility. But I know it now, and for as long as I live,
Spider-Man will never shirk his duty again. Robbers,
killers, beware. Spider-Man is here.

★ all quotes from Paul Soles as Spider-Man in *Spider-Man*

The Incredible Hulk *(1978–1982)*
Stars: Lou Ferrigno, Bill Bixby, Jack Colvin

Another Marvel Comics teen favorite is *The Incredible Hulk*, Dr. David
Bruce Banner (Bill Bixby), who as a result of a nuclear military accident,
turns into a supersize green monster whenever someone gets on his nerves.
The Hulk (Lou Ferrigno) spends his episodic life fleeing from the military
father who created and now seeks to destroy him. In his downtime, Hulk
struggles to gain control of his strange power and direct his nuclear rage
toward positive ends. The Hulk appeals to the terrible teen in all of us
because he has no choice but to express his inner rage and enforce his will
to power, and somehow manages to live to tell about it in the morning.

HULKISMS

Hulk smash! Hulk bash! Hulk crash!

★ Lou Ferrigno as the Hulk in *The Incredible Hulk*

For six months I've been dragging myself to the gym, and for what? Now look at me. Jane Fonda can't crack concrete like this girl can.

★ Lisa Zane as the She-Hulk in *The Incredible Hulk*

Ain't it clear? Gamma is a girl's best friend.

★ Lisa Zane as the She-Hulk in *The Incredible Hulk*

You don't know what it's like to be a monster!

★ Lou Ferrigno as the Hulk in *The Incredible Hulk*

★ all quotes from the 1996–1997 animated series

SO NICE THEY DID IT TWICE

The Incredible Hulk (*1996–1997*)
Stars: Neal McDonough, Lou Ferrigno, Lisa Zane

It seems America just couldn't get enough of the green monster, and in 1982 and again in the mid-1990s, the animated version appeared in family rooms everywhere featuring the Hulk as a brute so savage that he made Lou Ferrigno's live-action Hulk look like a slightly irritated commuter by comparison. The animated Hulk could smash cars, toss planes, and send ballistic missiles flying with a flick of his wrist. The animated series had the added benefit of Jennifer Walters and her alter ego, She-Hulk, who could match the Hulk blow for blow. If you're in the mood for a truly hard-core Hulkathon, check out this action-packed cartoon celebrating the teen beast within.

Batman *(1966–1968)*
*Stars: Adam West, Burt Ward, Lee Meriwether, Cesar
Romero, Burgess Meredith, Frank Gorshin, Julie
Newmar*

Batman (Adam West), the caped crusader, and his boy wonder, Robin (Burt Ward) (hmm…), live among us, virtually unnoticed, as the unassuming and wealthy entrepreneur Bruce Wayne and his ward, Dick Grayson (hmm…). But when night falls, Bruce and Dick don black leather masks and capes too, and really macho-looking utility belts, complete with crampons, hydraulics, and a virtual pharmacy of designer bat-drugs. And then they slide down a pole and descend into their bat cave, where they make a lot of frantic calls on their hotline, and then climb into their convertible Batmobile and head for Gotham City to seek out the forces of evil (hmmm…). What they usually come up with is Eartha Kitt or Julie Newmar in a catsuit, or the Joker (Cesar Romero), an aging and inebriated miscreant who laughs at his own bad jokes and wears way too much red lipstick. And while this sounds like a relatively normal mix of people to encounter on any given midnight in some inner teen-friendly sections of Gotham City, Batman is resolved to wipe out this sort of local color, because Batman is actually very prim and proper, and cultured underneath all that black leather. And he knows a lot about vintage wine, and exotic foods, and tasteful table decorations. And I think we'll just leave it right there, rather than go any further into the meat market district of this particular brand of hero worship, because this is, after all, a chapter for inner teens. But take it from us, when it comes to marvels, Batman is packing.

YOUR FREUDIAN SLIP IS SHOWING

I'm just going to hang around the bar. I don't want to look conspicuous.
★ Adam West as Batman in *Batman*

I'll be back in three minutes and twenty seconds.
★ Adam West as Batman in *Batman*

Holy atomic pile, Batman!
★ Burt Ward as Robin in *Batman*

Robin, warm up the Bat-spot analyzer while I take a sample of this affected cloth.
★ Adam West as Batman in *Batman*

Holy priceless collection of Etruscan snoods!
★ Burt Ward as Robin in *Batman*

Just a second while I retrieve my beanie, my hair, my tweezers, and my notes.
★ Adam West as Batman in *Batman*

I've just perfected an electronic hair Bat-analyzer, which may hold the key to this baffling question.
★ Adam West as Batman in *Batman*

Under this garb, we're perfectly ordinary Americans.
★ Burt Ward as Robin in *Batman*

■ *Saved by the Bell (1989–1993)*
   Stars: Mario López, Mark-Paul Gosselaar, Elizabeth Berkley,
      Tiffani Thiessen (before the Amber days), Lark Voorhies,
      Dennis Haskins, Dustin Diamond

Before they all grew into B-list careers, these *Saved by the Bell* kids were the students of Bayside High. This show focuses on the six major stereotypes in your basic high school.

There's the dork, the stud, the athlete, the prom queen, the straight-A student, the obligatory ethnic student, and the supergeek who talks real funny and who is accepted by the in-crowd because he makes everybody laugh. Let's face it, this was never a masterpiece of television writing. It has that after-school-special aftertaste, and the kids are never even remotely plausible. But there is just something soothing to the inner geek about watching Elizabeth Berkley and Mario López in their Mouseketeer phase really stinking up the joint. So when you're feeling left out of the "in-group" in your life, spend some time at Bayside, where everyone is in, because everyone is out.

LIVE TO TAPE

Saved by the Bell was originally a show called *Good Morning, Ms. Bliss* that debuted on Disney and was then canceled, but was saved by the bell when NBC picked it up.

DISASTERTHERAPY

Rich Girls *(2003)*
Stars: Ally Hilfiger, Jaime Gleicher, Tommy Hilfiger

This short-lived but very refreshing series follows two of New York's richest girls, Ally Hilfiger, designer Tommy Hilfiger's daughter, and her best friend, Jaime Gleicher, as they spend the last year of high school at the tony Dalton School on Manhattan's Upper East Side. And yet despite all of their privilege and designer élan, they are still awkward adolescents.

We watch transfixed as Ally and Jaime ride a roller coaster of extreme emotions as they try to execute the Herculean tasks of teendom, like finding an outfit for graduation or building a burrito. The feelings of failure that arise out of these trivial rites of passage cause the girls to go into shame spirals that can only be cured by a jaunt to the Caribbean or a week in a Zen spa somewhere on the other side of the international dateline. And when they come back . . . they are *still* awkward adolescents. When you're at an awkward stage, there is something indescribably delicious about watching two girls who have everything suddenly realizing that all the money in the world can't make you cool, only maturity can.

CHAPTER 6

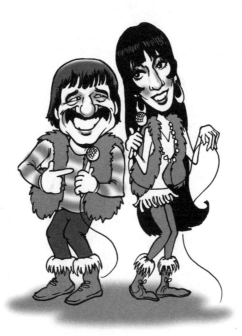

Codependent TV

IF YOU'VE BEEN UNLUCKY in love and are in the mood for a little TV and sympathy, retreat to your corner, sit out a few rounds, and let one of these codependent TV couples battle it out for you. These shows feature the best and the worst in TV twosomes and will remind you that as bad as things get, there is always somebody out there who can make a worse mess of things than you have—and besides, after a fight with your partner, there is nothing better than a little make-up TV.

▪ *Nip/Tuck (2003–)*
  Stars: *Dylan Walsh, Julian McMahon, John Hensley, Valerie Cruz,*
    Joely Richardson

When you're in the mood for a codependent feast, and ready to indulge in some good old-fashioned masochism, go under the knife with the codependent cutters of *Nip/Tuck*, who attempt to cure their self-esteem issues with a scalpel and invariably wind up nicking a vital organ or two in the process, escalating the situation from cosmetic to code blue.

Doctors Sean MacNamara (Dylan Walsh) and Christian Troy (Julian McMahon) are best friends and partners in a Miami-based plastic surgery practice where they lift the faces, tuck the tummies, and enlarge the breasts of an unending stream of lost and flawed souls in search of a quick fix to deeply buried psychic infections that a surgeon's knife could never even approach, let alone lance. And in a classic example of physicians who really need to heal themselves, our enabling surgeons persist in prescribing and dispensing their fantasy of perfection, as if beauty were a panacea that could cure everything from repressed abuse memories to the Oedipal syndrome.

This show is one big metaphor for what can happen when you try and fix huge problems by changing the mere appearance of things, and reminds us all that true change requires a little digging, because genuine love and happiness are much more than skin deep.

WORDS TO LIVE BY

The line that divides the porn industry and plastic surgery is a thin one.
We're both selling fantasy, aren't we?
  ★ Julian McMahon as Dr. Christian Troy in *Nip/Tuck*

You really want to get inside a woman? Stop thinking like a dick.
  ★ Roma Maffia as Liz Winters in *Nip/Tuck*

I'd rather be a good doctor who helps people than a brilliant doctor who hurts them.
  ★ Dylan Walsh as Sean McNamara in *Nip/Tuck*

▪ *Newlyweds: Nick & Jessica (2003–)*
  Stars: Jessica Simpson, Nick Lachey

This reality show chronicling the first year in the marriage between two picture-perfect pop stars, Nick Lachey and Jessica Simpson, is like what would have happened if Ricky Ricardo finally let Lucy in the show, and she wound up touring the country playing to stadium crowds while Ricky sat home with Fred doing interviews about Lucy's babbaloo and paying for his own lunch at the club. Needless to say, the garden path has a few thorns in this up-close look at new marriage between two people who have everything, including each other.

This reality show was originally intended to follow up MTV's success with *The Osbournes*, only in this series we watch a pop-star couple, as opposed to a heavy-metal family, as they work through the mundane details of day-to-day life, to see if family life really is greener on the other side of the celebrity fence. And ironically, where *The Osbournes* are concerned, we discover that even if you're an aging rocker who once bit the head off of a rodent for publicity, family life still looks pretty much like family life, once you get past the shock wigs, tattoos, and prescription pain medication.

What we discover with Nick and Jessica, though, is surprisingly the exact opposite: once you get past the Da Vinci veneers, the carefully sculpted abs, the double-knit catsuits, and all that hair, what you find are the spinning wheels of a sinister conspiracy theory, which can make even Mouseketeers into unwitting monsters in a corporate scheme to turn us all into McMansion-dwelling, remote-controllable consumers who always buy brand names and wear *a lot* of suede.

When you're feeling like your happily ever after doesn't look like it did in the fairy tales, let Nick and Jessica remind you that Disney can't buy you love, that people who have everything also have problems, and that even pop stars poop.

JESSICA'S JAW DROPPERS

I have bubbles in my tummy . . . it's just air. It's not stink. Promise.

Is that weird, taking my Louis Vuitton bag camping?

I have to go . . . drop some kids in the pool.

Is this chicken or is this fish? I know it's tuna. But it says chicken. By the sea.

★ all quotes from Jessica Simpson on *Newlyweds: Nick & Jessica*

■ *The Honeymooners (1955–1956)*
Stars: Jackie Gleason, Art Carney, Audrey Meadows, Joyce Randolph

This surefire cure for the codependent blues stars the great one, Jackie Gleason, as Ralph Kramden, a down-on-his-luck bus driver in Bed-Stuy, Brooklyn, who dreams of a bigger and better life once his ship finally comes in. Together with his best friend, Ed Norton (Art Carney), a sewer worker whose brains have gone a little soggy, he cooks up scheme after scheme to catapult himself over the harbor.

The hole in Ralph's sail is his steadfast first mate, Alice (Audrey Meadows), the salt of his earth, who always warns Ralph that his boat won't float before the water gets too deep, and matches him, bang for zoom, through every swell and trough of love American style in the 1950s. In addition to the reassurance that your significant other really does love you underneath all of that "bluster" about sending you to the moon, *The Honeymooners* is a comforting reminder that when it comes to the state of marriage in America, we really have come a long way, baby. The same, unfortunately, cannot be said of sitcoms. This one is a Gleason comedy classic!

RALPH AND ALICE'S BANG ZOOMS

Ralph: This is probably the biggest thing I ever got into.
Alice: The biggest thing you ever got into was your pants.

Ralph: Yessir, this is the time I'm gonna get my pot of gold.
Alice: Just go for the gold, you've already got the pot.

Ralph: What I say goes.
Alice: Then you better say "Alice" because I'm going.

Alice: Maybe you won't have to get the margarine, Trix. Four hundred
pounds of lard just walked in.

Ralph: You have just said the secret word, Alice. You have just
won a trip to the moon.

Ralph: One of these days Alice, bang zoom!
★ all quotes by Jackie Gleason as Ralph and Audrey Meadows as Alice
in *The Honeymooners*

▪ *The Sonny and Cher Show* (1976–1977)
Stars: Sonny Bono, Cher

The Sonny and Cher Show is like an updated version of *The Honeymooners* and is a really good cure for the my-true-love-is-tardy blues. This series, which ran only briefly and also, like *The Honeymooners*, to much popular acclaim, dissolved along with Sonny and Cher's relationship. And it's no wonder. Because this wasn't 1955, but the seventies, when people really should have known better than to dress up domestic dissolution in Bob Mackie gowns, set it to music, and put it on the air as a prime-time comedy/variety show for family audiences. This is the kind of stuff that nuptial nightmares are made of, and is a great reminder that just because two people are singing together doesn't make it harmony.

STRANGE BEDFELLOWS

Because TV can make for some couples that are out of this world.

Mork and Mindy (1978–1982)
Stars: Robin Williams, Pam Dawber

In his debut TV vehicle, Robin Williams stars as the man/child/alien Mork, a seventies-style ET come to earth in rainbow suspenders to study earthlings and report back to his native planet, Ork, on human behavior. Fortunately, Mork winds up living in Boulder, Colorado, in the seventies, where everybody looks like a refugee from a *Godspell* tour, so nobody much noticed the alien in their midst. Mork winds up sharing an apartment in the student district with an Ivory Girl in Birkenstocks who's living life day by day. On the outside, Mindy (Pam Dawber) is the picture of good health, happiness, and self-confidence. But secretly, Mindy despairs that she will never find her Mr. Right and become the ideal eighties-style wife and mom she's always dreamed of becoming, restoring a Victorian home and raising socially aware kids.

Fortunately for Mindy, she is saved from her fate by a visitor from outer space and beamed up to a future she never envisioned for herself. Yes, the Ivory Girl falls for her space creature, who is really just a big and extremely loquacious metaphor for arrested male development, as apparently everybody ages backward on Ork. The guy even sleeps in an egg, for God's sake. It's not like seventies sitcom symbolism could ever be called super subtle. But Mindy and her perpetually prepubescent alien were definitely a couple of the strangest bedfellows to ever nano-nano on network TV, and with taste in men like that, it's no wonder that Mindy eventually turned into Sam, living in San Francisco with her sister.

Bewitched *(1964–1972)*
Stars: Elizabeth Montgomery, Dick York, Dick Sergeant, Agnes Moorhead, Erin Murphy, Alice Pearce, Paul Lynde

Unbeknownst to his coworkers and friends, mild-mannered ad exec Darren Stevens's (Dick York/Dick Sergeant) trophy wife, Samantha (Elizabeth Montgomery), is actually a witch with magical powers who can do stuff like turn her husband into an inanimate object or make the china fly with a tiny twitch of her nose. And the worst part is, so can her mother. And while Samantha is happy to try and live with the promise she made along with her marriage vows never to use her magical powers again, her mother, Endora (Agnes Moorhead), who is a lot like Auntie Mame with Bette Davis eyes, has other ideas, and tortures her mortal son-in-law with everything she's got in her considerable arsenal.

Darren and Samantha, and later their witchy daughter, Tabitha (Erin Murphy), are living the American dream in this split-level, suburban ranch-style Salem while the powerful crone looms in the background, mouthing the matriarchal wisdom of the ages, and reminding her daughter that it's not nice to fool Mother Nature. This is perhaps one of the quirkiest metaphors for codependence ever produced on TV.

ENDORA'S EPITHETS

Samantha, I will not stand here and be insulted by something which is 94 percent water.

Don't talk to your mother like that. I'll tell you when you're happy.

Dishwashers…women's clubs…freeways…I'd be frightened to death too.

That's a human being for you; spend most of their lives running in circles for a series of nothing.

★ all quotes from Agnes Moorhead as Endora in *Bewitched*

I Dream of Jeannie *(1965–1970)*
Stars: Barbara Eden, Larry Hagman, Bill Daily, Hayden Rorke

Major Nelson (Larry Hagman) is an astronaut who, while on a secret covert ops mission for NASA, finds a bottle with a genie inside. Once freed, the genie named Jeannie (Barbara Eden) is so thrilled that she pledges to serve Master Nelson for the rest of her life, granting every one of his wishes, even the really stupid ones, and always, always showing up for her genie shift wearing a belly shirt, harem pants, and a Chanel-inspired fez with a pink chiffon chin strap, which is half Jackie O. and half damsel in distress. Yet despite the medieval premise of this show, and this TV union, Jeannie, much like Samantha Stevens, has special powers that allow her to keep her master in check whenever he gets out of line. And like the Stevenses, this ideal sixties man must keep his woman's power a secret from his neighbors and employers. Well, harem pants and belly shirts wouldn't come into fashion for another fifteen years, and neither would women who are more powerful than their masters.

▪ Moonlighting *(1985–1989)*
Stars: Cybill Shepherd, Bruce Willis, Allyce Beasley

This tongue-in-cheek TV interpretation of a Bogie and Bacall movie features an eighties-style self-conscious narrator, a flair for scathingly funny one-liners, and one of the most mismatched couples ever to throw the book at one another on network TV. Maddie Hayes (Cybill Shepherd), a former supermodel (of course she is; this was the eighties, after all), is betrayed by her manager and left with nothing except a half-bankrupt detective agency, headed by David Addison (Bruce Willis), a Sam Spade knockoff with a rakish grin and macho mischievousness that he wears on his face like a five o'clock shadow. The only problem is, Maddie is as much a man as David, and every week they battle it out to determine who is the most macho, and somehow, Maddie wins hands down every single time.

HE SAID, SHE SAID

Just when I think you've gone as low as you can go, you find a basement door!

★ Cybill Shepherd as Maddie Hayes in *Moonlighting*

Boy, are you a tough customer. I bet you didn't even clap your hands to save Tinkerbell.

★ Bruce Willis as David Addison in *Moonlighting*

Bev's TV Tray

If you're looking for a recipe to put the fun back in your dysfunctional relationship, try out this three-course canoodle feast guaranteed to set you both on the path toward happily ever after. This menu is simple, easy to prepare, and rich in opportunities to eat with your fingers, and will create sensuous memories that will linger long after the boys of summer have gone.

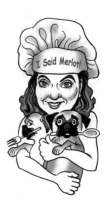

Naked Oysters

Just pry them open and lay them on a platter of ice; if you're a strict nudist, squeeze a little lemon juice on them. Otherwise you can accessorize your oysters with minced horseradish, cocktail sauce, or a hot pepper vinaigrette. Then pick up the shell, slide the thing in your mouth, and swallow it all down without thinking about it too much.

Afterglow Penne

Just one lovin' spoonful of this pulchritudinous pasta and you'll understand why so many codependent romances are set in Tuscany.

Here's what you'll need:
1 pound penne
3 tablespoons olive oil
1 sweet Italian sausage
2 red bell peppers
2 yellow bell peppers
3 cioppino onions
1 bulb diced fennel, white part sliced
2 cloves garlic
Salt, pepper, oregano, basil
1 cup chicken broth
$^{1}/_{2}$ pound fresh smoked mozzarella, cubed

Here's how you do it:
Cook penne al dente in a lot of water, a tablespoon of olive oil, and a pinch of salt. Drain and set aside. Boil sausage in a saucepan in water that barely covers the sausage. Let all the water boil away (along with the fat) and leave the pan on until the sausages have browned. Cut sausage into thin slices. Heat a little olive oil in a large skillet and sauté peppers, onions, fennel, garlic, and seasonings. Cook until garlic is clear, then remove the garlic and add the chicken broth. Simmer for 2 to 3 minutes. Add the sausage slices and pasta to the sautéed vegetables. Finally, toss in the cubed smoked mozzarella, a little more olive oil, salt, and pepper and stir until just heated through. Put it in a big bowl and serve without forks.

The Simultaneous Orgasm
(Satisfies 2)
For dessert, both of you can take a bite of this chocolate soufflé at the same time and experience the heights of culinary bliss.

Here's what you'll need:
2 tablespoons butter, melted
6 tablespoons sugar
1 cup milk
2 ounces semisweet chocolate
3 tablespoons cocoa powder
$\frac{1}{2}$ cup flour
$\frac{1}{4}$ cup butter, softened
$\frac{1}{4}$ cup powdered sugar
4 egg yolks
5 egg whites
Chocolate sauce

Here's how you do it:
Preheat oven to 400°F. Grease a soufflé dish with melted butter and dust with 6 tablespoons granulated sugar. Next, combine milk and chocolate in a saucepan. Add cocoa powder and bring to a boil, stirring constantly. Make a paste with the flour, butter, and powdered sugar and add it gradually to the boiling milk. Next, whisk in the egg yolks and cook until mixture is creamy and begins to thicken. In a bowl whisk the egg whites until stiff and fold into the custard. Fill the soufflé dish to within $\frac{1}{2}$ inch of the top and place in a pan in 3 to 4 inches of hot water. Bake in preheated oven for 40 minutes. When a butter knife stuck into the center comes out clean, it's done. Serve with a warm chocolate sauce on top. The rest should be self-explanatory.

▪ *I Love Lucy* (1951–1957)
Stars: Lucille Ball, Desi Arnaz, Vivian Vance, William Frawley

Zany fifties housewife Lucy Ricardo (Lucille Ball) wants nothing more than to be a big star and share the limelight with her Cuban bandleader husband, Ricky Ricardo (Desi Arnaz). Unfortunately, Lucy has no talent whatsoever, and Ricky, regardless, isn't too anxious to encourage his wife's aspirations. This forms the basis for six years of groundbreaking comedy, featuring the battle between Ricky and Lucy that held America on the edge of its collective couch, waiting to see what kind of trouble Lucy would get into next, and how she would "'splain" the mess to Ricky. *I Love Lucy* is an uplifting reminder that despite the unfulfilled dreams that we all may have, the love of your friends and a partner who understands you, even though he may not speak the language too well, is all that heaven allows.

LUCY'S GOOSEYS

Ever since we said "I do," there have been so many things that we don't.

Yeah, he's pushing twenty-three all right. He's pushed it all the way to thirty-five.

I'd just love a Richard Widmark grapefruit to go with my Robert Taylor orange.... What a fruit salad that would make.

The next time you want hamburgers without onions, ask for hamburgers without onions. Don't stand there and yell, "Bring the bull in the ring and laugh in his face!"

★ all from Lucille Ball as Lucy Ricardo in *I Love Lucy*

LIVE TO TAPE

Desi Arnaz was a real bandleader, who single-handedly launched the conga craze in the United States. When Lucy was approached about doing the show, the producers didn't want Desi to play her husband because he was Latin, so Lucy and Desi took back the show and created Desilu Productions so that they could have creative control. While Lucy was often considered the star and the powerhouse behind their success, in fact, Desi pioneered many techniques that made the American sitcom what it is today. Among his innovations are the filming of TV shows with multiple cameras, taping in front of a live audience, using a warm-up man before taping, and reruns.

WHY CAN'T WE BE FRIENDS?

It's kind of ironic that some of the most functional couples on TV aren't really couples at all, but "just friends." Then again, given the complexity of sexual politics in America, perhaps it's understandable why TV would avoid the drama altogether, or maybe they're trying to tell us that best friends make the best marriages.

- *Will & Grace (1998–)*
  Stars: Debra Messing, Eric McCormack, Sean Hayes, Megan Mullally

The setup for this NBC hit series is a lot like what might have happened if Mary in *The Mary Tyler Moore Show* had moved into her charming restored Victorian with her gay best friend. Or if Mary was a Mary. When Grace (Debra Messing) and Will (Eric McCormack) go through bad breakups, they move in together in a charming apartment in New York City and keep each other codependently happy until the real thing comes along. They are surrounded by a coterie of friends, most notably Karen Walker (Megan Mullally), Grace's unpaid assistant who works just to kill time and who is rather like Dorothy Parker with a better bustline and a state-of-the-art pharmacist, and "Just Jack" (Sean Hayes), Will's flamboyantly gay friend who is in love with Cher, show tunes, and himself, although not necessarily in that order.

Along with a rotating cast of celebrity guests, including Madonna, Cher (of course), J-Lo, Gregory Hines, Sydney Pollack, Debbie Reynolds, and Molly Shannon, *Will & Grace* asks us a very good question…what's wrong with codependence if it works? And while Will and Grace may not always be able to answer that question, and may never find the "real thing" that they're waiting for in each other, they nevertheless support each other unconditionally, respect each other as individuals, and most important, remember that love is love is love is love.

HE SAID, SHE SAID

Grace: Okay, here's the Thanksgiving menu so far: apple pie, pumpkin pie, blueberry tart, and ice-cream roll. What am I missing? Cake. We need cake.
Will: Did you take a bong hit before you wrote that?

Will: Look at this. I'll bet Courtney Love has probably peed in this very toilet.
Grace: Or, at the very least, around it.

Grace: Look, my choices were flawless, and if your client can't see that, then he is guilty of extremely bad taste, and isn't that the real crime here today?

Will: Gracie, there is no—
Grace: Objection. The familiar cutening of my name implies we like each other.

Will: Your dad's great.
Grace: Yeah, in a parallel universe where my hair is straight and so are you.
★   all quotes from Eric McCormack as Will and Debra Messing as
Grace in *Will & Grace*

▪ *The Odd Couple (1970–1975)*
Stars: Tony Randall, Jack Klugman

Never was there a more unlikely TV couple than Felix Unger (Tony Randall) and Oscar Madison (Jack Klugman), two divorced guys thrown together when their wives kick them out, who are for some reason determined to make a life together even though they are completely mismatched.

Oscar is a sloppy sportswriter who lives on hot dogs and beer, thinks Pavarotti is a kind of pasta, and never, ever cleans his room. Felix is a hypochondriacal, neat freak "fashion photographer" (hint, hint) who lives for merlot and Mozart and always cleans his room. Episode after episode, these two opposites who attract battle it out between clean and messy, gourmet and garage, and in the process, try to answer the central question of the series: Can two divorced men live together without driving each other crazy? And surprisingly, even though this was the seventies, the answer for *The Odd Couple* is yes.

Ironically, this show, which depended upon divorce as a premise, is one of the best TV lessons we've seen on how to have a functional relationship. Oscar and Felix clash, but they ultimately respect and love each other as individuals, and don't expect each other to change. Even though they are different, they are the same in their bond of mutual love and respect for each other, and end up becoming one of the most memorable couples in TV history.

So if you've been fighting with your other half about who didn't do his or her share around the house, put down that frying pan, pick up your remote, and spend a few hours with *The Odd Couple* together, and let Oscar and Felix remind you that love means never having to say it's your turn to do the dishes.

HE SAID, HE SAID

Oscar: You want brown juice or green juice?
Felix: What's the difference?
Oscar: Three weeks.

Oscar: *You ruined my wine.*
Felix: *Here's a dollar. Buy another three bottles.*

Felix: *What do you dream about?*
Oscar: *Living alone.*

Oscar: *That's fun fat. Everybody has that.*
Felix: *I don't.*
Oscar: *You don't have any fun, either.*

★　all quotes from Jack Klugman as Oscar Madison and Tony Randall as
Felix Unger in *The Odd Couple*

■ *Laverne & Shirley (1976–1983)*
　Stars: Penny Marshall, Cindy Williams, Michael McKean,
　　David L. Lander

Laverne DeFazio (Penny Marshall) and Shirley Feeney (Cindy Williams), two pink-slipped bottle cappers from the Schotz Brewery in Milwaukee, Wisconsin, eventually lose their jobs and head to Burbank to find their dreams of a new life and new loves. And while they, like Felix and Oscar, are something of an odd couple (Laverne is Oscar, Shirley is Felix), they are nevertheless able to overcome their stylistic differences and love and support each other unconditionally for the better part of eight seasons, not to mention develop a long-term romance with syndication. Together with their male counterparts on the show—Lenny (Michael McKean) and Squiggy (David L. Lander), two stooges who like Laverne and Shirley are together wherever they go—they teach us all that no matter where you go, there you are, which is okay as long as you're there with your partner.

SHE SAID, SHE SAID

Shirley: Someday, God willing, I'm gonna be a mother. And if my daughter comes to me and says, Mama, I want to go to this bachelor party and come outta this cake...what can I tell her?
Laverne: A lot more than most mothers!
★ Penny Marshall as Laverne and Cindy Williams as Shirley in
Laverne & Shirley

SHAKING HANDS WITH THE MONSTER

These extreme makeover shows remind us of all the amazing stuff we can do when we work together.

Monster Garage *(2002–2005)*
Jesse James, who *is* related, assembles a crew of garage geeks and maverick mechanics and together they transform ordinary vehicles into fabulous Mad Max–inspired monster machines. Their motto is make it loud and make it cool. They have just seven days to complete these miracles of the motorway, and usually a limited budget, and must rely on teamwork, Jesse's leadership, and their own imagination and resourcefulness to create the ultimate highway Hannibal that will eat up the road.

In each episode the team must decide on a plan, agree on a budget, and then set to work hammering, hoisting, and hemming and hawing while some really cheesy cheerleaders root them on from the wings as they put the *wreck* in *recreational.* In the end, innocent Esplanades, Beetles, and Lincolns are transformed into vehicles designed for purposes straight out of your wildest gearhead fantasies, and equipped with options that Henry Ford never dreamed of, like suicide doors, hatchback barbecues, monster grilles, or something called a kegerator. This is a show about baggy jeans and beer, tattoos and tailgates, rims and routers, and most of all, it's about teamwork, and a great reminder for the gearhead in your life that people skills are as important as routers when it comes to building a dream.

Monster House (2003–)

This spin-off of *Monster Garage* brings together a group of five or six renovation renegades, male and female, and together they turn some poor, unsuspecting bugger's humble abode into a monster house custom-made to remind us that it takes more than four walls and a roof to make a home. There must also be a Brazilian-inspired air tub delivery system to transport beer from the kitchen to the living room. And a casino.

Like its parent show, *Monster House* is more about the journey than the destination, and watching these mismatched construction teams struggling to beat the clock without beating up each other is a big part of the payoff. It reminds us all that no one is an island, no matter what you can do with your own two hands.

CHAPTER 7

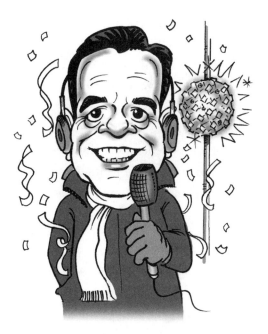

Party TV

TV IS NOT ONLY good company when you're alone, it's also a way to share quality time with friends and family, by sharing the memorable TV moments that we all have in common. Whether it's the start of the new season of *American Idol*, Ross and Rachel's wedding, or last call at *Cheers*, it's great to invite over the main characters in your life, mix up a batch of cocktails, whip up a holiday spread, and watch TV history being made, together.

- *American Idol (2000–)*
  Stars: Simon Cowell, Paula Abdul, Randy Jackson, Ryan Seacrest

What better reason to throw a party than America's search for the next pop icon? Three judges, thousands of young hopefuls, countless ballads, and one overly excited host make for a fun night to hang with the aspiring superstars in your life and dream about your moments in the sun.

American Idol, the *Star Search* for a new millennium, pits unknown singers from across the country against one another in a talent contest to find America's next big phenom. But while it's always fun to watch Kelly or Reuben or Clay vying for the top slot, it's even better party fodder to watch the losers, like William Hung, who don't let a small detail like an absolute lack of musical talent get in the way of their pop-star dreams. Until of course the scathing talent judge Simon Cowell lays a few of his powerful similes on them. So the next time you're throwing a bash for a new generation of glitterati, put *American Idol* on mute in the background and turn it up when William Hung hits the flat screen. Then raise a glass with your favorite celebrity hopefuls to dreams coming true, because if it happened to William Hung, it could happen to you.

SIMON SAYS

You look like a pen salesman, and you have the personality of a mouse.

You and salsa go together like chocolate ice cream and an onion.

My advice would be if you want to pursue a career in the music business, don't.

*Did you really believe you could become the American Idol?
Well, then, you're deaf.*

*If you would have been singing like this two thousand years ago,
people would have stoned you.*

*If your lifeguard duties were as good as your singing, a lot of
people would be drowning.*

★ all quotes from Simon Cowell in *American Idol*

▪ *The Super Bowl*

There's no TV bonding experience quite like getting together with that old gang of yours on Super Sunday and rooting for the home team while consuming as much fat, salt, sugar, and carbonated hops as you can get your hands on without spraining something. Super Bowl Sunday parties—which began when the Green Bay Packers inaugurated the Super Bowl games by beating the Kansas City Chiefs back in 1967—are as American as apple pie or SUVs or aggressive foreign policies.

But even if you're not a sports fan, there's lots of great ways to enjoy the Super Bowl with friends. The halftime show is always great camp fare, as Janet Jackson can definitely attest, and the commercials, which are the most expensive spots all year, often pack more punch than either of the offensive lines on the field. And then, of course, there's the food. So if you need a little pep in your pom-poms, try throwing a Super Bowl Sunday party this year and score a TV touchdown, no matter which team wins.

Bev's TV Tray: Super Bowl Taco Mousse

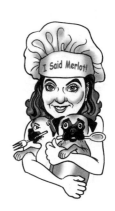

This classic Super Bowl snack comes to me via my sports-addicted friend Kim Doi, whose sister Angie Donaldson serves this recipe whenever the Chiefs play, because something in the room has to score.

Here's what you'll need:
One 16-ounce can refried beans
8 ounces cream cheese, softened
1 cup sour cream, plus extra for garnish
2 tablespoons taco seasoning
2 garlic cloves, pressed
½ cup (2 ounces) shredded cheddar cheese
One medium tomato, seeded and diced

4 green onions, white parts thinly sliced
¹/₂ cup sliced black olives
2 tablespoons finely chopped fresh cilantro
1 tablespoon Frank's hot sauce
Dash nutmeg
Tortilla chips

Here's how you do it:
Preheat oven to 350 degrees. Spread beans over bottom of an oiled baking dish. Combine cream cheese, sour cream, taco seasoning, hot sauce, and garlic. Mix well. Spread over beans. Sprinkle shredded cheese on top. Bake 15 to 20 minutes or until cheese is melted. Sprinkle tomato, onions, olives, and cilantro over dip. Garnish with additional sour cream, if desired. Serve with tortilla chips.

BROADWAY TV

■ *The Annual Tony Awards*

Once a year, musical theater's best step out from behind the footlights and in front of the cameras to toast Broadway. What better excuse is there than the Tony Awards to invite over the show-tune queens in your life and have a Great White Way-athon?

The best place to see the fashion, music, and politics that are affecting us is at this annual choreographed recap of the best that Forty-second Street's got to offer each season. Whether it's Betty Buckley dressed as an old Jellicle Cat belting out the 10 o'clock number while rising up to heaven on a tire engulfed in billows of stage smoke, or Glenn Close as an aging silent screen diva whose monstrous ego murders her young lover, or Nathan Lane and Matthew Broderick purposely producing a Broadway flop, the Tonys always deliver a double helping of the fabulous and the grotesque and let us all recapture a little bit of the magic even if we don't have front-row seats. So call in your cast, shake some 'tinis, and celebrate the latest and the greatest lullabies of Broadway.

■ *Broadway: The American Musical* (2004)
Director: Michael Kantor

This six-part PBS special, hosted by Julie "four octaves" Andrews (who else?), showcases over one hundred years of musical theater, from the bawdy vaudevillian utopias of *The Ziegfeld Follies* to the alternative Oz in *Wicked*. Michael Kantor takes us behind the red curtain and immerses us in all of the multitudinous details that go into the making of a Broadway hit. We're shown everything from how the writers and composers create their story to the vision of the director and designers to the high-stakes gamble taken by the producers. No song is left unsung, no sequin unsewn in this comprehensive special custom-made for the theater fanatic. This makes a great warm-up act for your next Tony Awards gathering.

PAGEANT TV

Haven't you heard? Pageants are not really an anachronistic and often macabre display of the superficial values placed on women in a consumer-driven society. They're a scholarship contest. So the next time the crown is up for grabs, dust off your tiara, get the girls together, and throw a pageant bash and celebrate the sisterhood, because as all inner beauty queens know, the crown goes to the gal who has the best friends.

Miss America

Tracing its origins back to the boardwalk in Atlantic City over seventy-five years ago, Miss America is the grandmother of all beauty pageants. Today, what began as "the Most Beautiful Bathing Girl in Atlantic City" contest, where the winner received a golden mermaid for her efforts, has become a nationally televised event, where contestants from across the land parade through our living rooms in evening gowns and swimsuits, and display their inner and outer talents for amateur critics. And while we will really miss the ventriloquism and the dramatic monologues and the arias now that they've eliminated the talent competition, there's still plenty of good clean camp to round out a girls' night, and make us all thankful that in our personal pageants, we don't have to simultaneously count calories and solve world hunger.

Miss Universe

What began as a bathing beauty contest sponsored by Catalina Swimwear in Long Beach, California, is now an annual international TV event bringing together beautiful humanitarians from around the world to compete for the coveted crown. This pageant features the same evening gowns and swimsuit competitions, but because it's a global beauty pageant, we also get a gander at all the gals in their traditional regional costumes. And while this pageant does present a unique opportunity to compare and contrast different cultural notions of beauty, the only distinction between these largely blonde global beauties is that Miss Holland usually sports a pair of wooden shoes at some point, while Miss India always dons a sari. Well, it is a Donald Trump production after all, and is therefore completely unafraid of its own tastelessness. So if you're in the mood for the hard stuff, *Miss Universe* is the pageant for you.

The Swan (2004)

Billed as the most unusual pageant ever devised, this reality competition gathers a gaggle of women who look like they've been having a bad-hair day for, like, decades, then turns them over to a team of TV surgeons, talk-show therapists, and network stylists who seem somewhat overly attached to their curling wands, and who transform these ducklings in sensible shoes into elegant swans in stilettos. In order to achieve the crown, these pageant contestants—most of whom look like they could be transformed with a hug, a reliable prescription for antidepressants, and a good sports bra—go under the knife, and after a few implants and veneers, liposuction, and dermabrasions, not to mention three months of recovery in a chin strap, emerge looking less like swans and more like a few of the soggier drag queens we saw down on Christopher Street last night. So the next time you're having an ugly-duckling moment, invite the whole gaggle over and tune in to *The Swan*, and be reminded that a smile is the best makeover there is and doesn't require stitches.

Bev's TV Tray: Beauty School Dropout's Pie

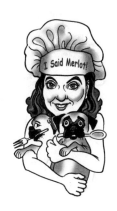

Because in order to experience true beauty you have to count your blessings, not your calories.

Here's what you'll need:
8 eggs
1¹/₂ cups milk
2 cups grated fresh mozzarella cheese
1 cup diced Parma ham or prosciutto
3 cups cooked spaghetti noodles
1 cup fresh diced tomatoes
Salt, pepper, and oregano to taste
1 cup grated Asiago cheese

Here's how you do it:
Preheat oven to 350 degrees. Beat eggs and milk until fluffy and light yellow in color. Stir in all remaining ingredients except the Asiago cheese and pour into a shallow baking pan. Sprinkle the Asiago over the top and bake covered with foil for 20 minutes, then uncover and bake for an additional 10 minutes until the eggs are done and the top is golden brown.

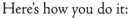

▪ *The Academy Awards*

What would the television universe be like without the Academy of Motion Pictures' star-studded annual salute to the movies that matter? Since its inception in 1929 we have counted on the Oscars to deliver hours and hours and hours of overlong and self-congratulatory, or gratuitously political, acceptance speeches, really horrendous production numbers, and the usual glittering coterie of stars who annually make their way up that legendary red carpet, and if we're lucky, fall off their heels or out of their designer fashion statements. What better way to celebrate with friends than with an Oscar bash and applaud our cinema sweethearts, boo at the celebrities we love to hate, and celebrate the movies that entertain us, define us, and give us something to talk about around the water cooler every morning. So whether it's been a year of musical comedy, big-screen epics, or gritty street dramas, invite your friends over for an Oscar bash and celebrate the stories that bind us.

OOPS, I SAID IT AGAIN

Billy Crystal: It was thirteen years ago when I first hosted the Academy Awards, and things sure have changed since then. George Bush was president, the economy was tanking, and we had just finished a war with Iraq. Yeah, things really have changed.

Denise Roberts: We're so thankful that The Lord of the Rings *did not qualify in this category.*

Cameron Diaz: For as long as the medium has existed the debate has raged: are movies art or entertainment? Well, how many movies these days are entertaining? Yes, movies are an art, but the person who directs this art that movies are, who was formerly called the art director, is now confusingly called the production designer. The production designer directs the work of the person currently called the art director and is himself usually a former art director who has gotten too big for his britches. But specifically, what does the production designer do? Well, he or she flits about the set, draping things and fabrics, hanging pictures on the wall, or if it's a World War II picture, arranging the mud. Everything you see on the screen except for the actors, who don't matter so much, is designed by the production designer, or if he didn't design it, he at least looked at it and said "Okay, we'll go with that." We honor, then, these strange artistic people.

Sally Field: You like me, you really like me.
★ all quotes from The Academy Awards

Danielle and Todd's Academy Award—Winning Punch

Try out this beauty of a punch at your next Oscar bash, and who knows? Maybe you'll wind up getting the award for the best offscreen romance!

Here's what you'll need:

1 empty half-gallon carton (it could be OJ, milk, or whatever you have available)

Pineapple juice and cranberry juice, blended

Lemons and/or limes

1 bottle of your favorite flavored vodka (I like raspberry)

2 bottles of your favorite inexpensive champagne (or sparkling wine)

Your favorite large bowl and ladle

Here's how you do it:

Okay, kids, this one is a little more involved, but it makes for a great punch that you won't have to do anything to all night. First rinse out your empty half-gallon carton, then siphon in your juice blend. It's up to you how tart or sweet you'd like it. I prefer to go to the more tart side if it's before a meal. Don't forget to squeeze in some lemon or lime to cut a little of the sweetness. Put on the lid and shake the hell out of it. Set it upright in your freezer (usually fits on the inside of the door). Do this the night before the party so you'll have a nice big ice cube of juices.

The next part is easy. Once your guests start to arrive, get out your juice cube and cut it out of the carton. Pour in the vodka (not too much; you want your guests to be able to get home alive!) and place your cube into the center of your punch bowl. Once there is a big enough group, you get to open the champagne! The main misconception is that you want a big pop when you open it. Wrong! If you do, your drink will have no bubbles and fall flat. Get a dish towel and firmly hold the cork with one hand and the bottom of the bottle with your other. The secret is to twist the bottle at the bottom and just hold the cork stationary.

Once you've eased out the cork, slowly pour your champagne over your ice cube so you can loosen some of the juice. Give a stir and serve! If you start running low, pop a second bottle and pour. Don't forget to make a toast to quality time with your closest circle of friends.

Note: the big secret with this punch is that the cube in the middle melts much slower than floating cubes would. Also, as it melts, it adds more punch to the mix, rather than the water normal ice cubes would add.

WHEN YOU NEED A LITTLE CHRISTMAS TV

If you're feeling like a Charlie in the Box, and Santa's rescue sled is still months away, invite your favorite misfit toys over to watch this trio of Christmas specials, guaranteed to deck your halls and fill you with the Christmas spirit, no matter what time of year.

Rudolph, the Red-Nosed Reindeer (1964)

Poor Rudolph. His friends laugh at him, he's not allowed to play in any reindeer games, even his family rejects him, and all because he has a funny nose. When the intolerance at the North Pole becomes unendurable, Rudolph, along with his fellow misfits, the elf/wannabe dentist Hermey and a perpetually unfortunate prospector, Cornelius, set out in search of more forgiving climes, only to run afoul of an abominable snowman with a bad overbite, and land on an entire island of misfit toys. Here at last these refugees from Toyland can feel like they belong. But when trouble brews back in Santa's workshop, only Rudolph can save the day, and we, along with all of the babes in Toyland, learn that when the fog gets thick, the only way to navigate the road ahead is to celebrate diversity and welcome everyone's unique gifts under the Christmas tree of life.

Hermey: Hey, what do you say we both be independent together, huh?
Rudolph: You wouldn't mind my red nose?
Hermey: Not if you don't mind me being a dentist.
Rudolph: It's a deal.
★ Paul Soles as Hermey and Billy Mae Richards as Rudolph in
Rudolph the Red-Nosed Reindeer

A Charlie Brown Christmas (1965)

Charlie Brown and Charles Schulz's whole fun cast decide to celebrate the holidays by putting on a pageant. Charlie Brown, although upset by the commercialism of Christmas, agrees to direct.

His first big task, to find the tree, falls short when he shows up with a limp pine branch. With a little love, a little faith, and a little help from his friends, not to mention a beautifully eloquent speech from Linus, who for once takes his thumb out of his mouth, Charlie's tree and his and our understanding of the true meaning of Christmas shine brightly through the long dark night.

Charlie Brown: Rats. Nobody sent me a Christmas card today. I almost wish there weren't a holiday season. I know nobody likes me. Why do we have to have a holiday season to emphasize it?
Lucy Van Pelt: I know how you feel about all this Christmas business, getting depressed and all that. It happens to me every year. I never get what I really want. I always get a lot of stupid toys or a bicycle or clothes or something like that.
Charlie Brown: What is it you want?
Lucy Van Pelt: Real estate.
★ Peter Robbins as Charlie Brown and Tracy Stratford as Lucy Van Pelt in
A Charlie Brown Christmas

How the Grinch Stole Christmas *(1966)*

The Grinch, who has a heart three sizes too small, lives in self-imposed exile in a cave on a hill, overlooking everybody having a much better time than he is down in Whoville. And as is usually the case in such situations, the Grinch starts to go green with malignant envy and devises a plot to vent his wrath on the poor but happy citizens below.

As Christmas approaches, the Grinch gets a brainstorm—he will steal Christmas. And sure enough, while the Whos down in Whoville are asleep in their Who beds, dreaming their Who Christmas dreams, in anticipation of a first-rate Who Christmas morning, the Grinch slithers in on tiptoe to steal the toys, the decorations, and even the roast beef. Yet despite all of this, the Whos wake up and still manage to have a good time, reminding the Grinch and all of us in the process that all you really need to have a good time at Christmas, or any other time of year, is love and kindness.

Welcome, Christmas, bring your cheer. Cheer to all Whos far and near.
Christmas Day is in our grasp so long as we have hands to clasp.
★ Boris Karloff as the narrator in *How the Grinch Stole Christmas*

ONE MORE FOR THE ROAD: FAREWELL TV

They say all good things come to an end, and with television shows, this proves to be really true. Once we start to watch our favorite shows religiously week after week, year after year, they become a part of our lives. We grow with the characters and talk about them as if we know them. So when the network pulls the plug, we must stand together, be strong, and mourn the loss of our TV favorites. So if you're looking for a reason to call up the old crew and relive the memories, try one of our final series farewells.

M*A*S*H Final Episode (1983)

"Goodbye, Farewell, and Amen"

*M*A*S*H*, which followed the lives of the members of the 4077th Mobile Army Surgical Hospital on the front lines in the Korean War, boasted a devoted and widespread audience. The series ran for eleven years, which is eight years longer than the Korean War lasted. When the final episode finally aired on February 28, 1983, 125 million people, the largest audience ever for a TV show, tuned in to say a tearful good-bye to Hawkeye, Hotlips, Radar, Klinger, and Hunnicut. Whether you were around to see this famous farewell broadcast or not, this is a poignant and compelling farewell to a band of TV brothers and sisters in arms, who taught us so many lessons about life, love, and most important, letting go.

Sex and the City Final Episode (2004)

"An American Girl in Paris (Part Deux)"

Sex and the City, which followed the love lives of four single girlfriends in the Big Bad Apple, finally threw us its final kiss on February 22, 2004. Four million of us tuned in to bid a fond bon voyage to Carrie, Samantha, Charlotte, and Miranda, who at last rode off into the sunset, having found true love at last. Carrie met her happily ever after wearing a $79,000 dress, of course. No wonder the final word of the final episode was *fabulous*. So when you're getting together with your kiss-and-tell buddies, put on your best designer rags, break out the Jimmy Choos, and say good night, ladies, over and over again to *Sex and the City* that never sleeps.

Friends Final Episode (2004)

"The Last One"

Friends, which followed the lives and loves of six lovable postadolescent caffeine achievers coming of age in, you guessed it, New York City, drank its final cup of joe on May 6, 2004. More than fifty-one million of us watched for one last time, as all of the loose ends were tied up in a neat bow. This series finale at last brought together our favorite couple who couldn't quite commit, gave Chandler and Monica, the couple who could commit but couldn't reproduce, twins, found Phoebe the perfect lid for her pot, and gave Joey a network deal. Who could ask for anything more? So when you're in the mood for a happy ending, invite your best friends over for a little latte and the finale of *Friends*, and raise a mug to life, love, exotic roasts, perennial adolescence, and friendship.

CHAPTER 8

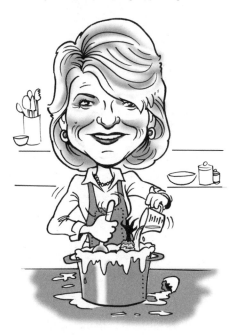

Antianxiety TV

WHEN YOU'VE BEEN WHITE-knuckling the armchair of life, let go with a little Antianxiety TV and relax your grip on the joystick of life. These shows—featuring some of television's most memorable control freaks, truth tellers, crusaders, and clowns—counsel us to face facts, laugh at our fears, and walk through the storm with our heads held high. Because the only thing to fear is fear itself . . . well, that and losing the remote control in the couch cushions.

▪ *The Awful Truth (1999–2000)*
   Stars: Michael Moore, Bruce Brown, Karen Duffy, Ben Hamper,
   Jay Martel, Jerry Minor, Katie Roberts

If you're feeling buffeted about by the winds of change and are longing to stick your head in the sand until the dust settles, let this series from Michael Moore, big champion of the little guy, remind you that it's always better to face the awful truth than have it sneak up and bite you in the bottom line.

In this guerrilla activist reality series, Moore takes his unrelenting lens into the board-rooms, theme parks, banks, and gas stations of America to uncover corruption and greed wherever they lurk. In each episode, Moore confronts corporate and political bullies by asking the tough questions and broadcasting the answers into the living rooms of America.

Despite the very serious issues that are at the core of every Michael Moore production, there are also plenty of laughs, as if Moore were trying to counsel us that no matter how dark the forces at hand, laughter and truth are always the best defenses. Episodes include a stunt campaign to elect a ficus tree to political office to underscore the absurdity of our electoral process. And the ficus actually wins! Moore also stages a Salem-style witch hunt at the height of Monica-gate, a traveling political mosh pit, and a mock gas station advertising the lowest prices "and that's no Shiite," which attracts a landslide of business despite its open admission that all profits go to Saddam Hussein. In a world that seems to grow bigger and more divided every day, Michael Moore's awful truth comforts us that one man really can make a difference through the awesome power of the punch line, and encourages us that the best antidote for anxiety is taking action.

MICHAEL'S MOTS

Librarians see themselves as the guardians of the First Amendment. You got a thousand Mother Joneses at the barricades! I love the librarians, and I am grateful for them!

Anytime you got the pope and the Dixie Chicks against you, your time is up.

.As we neared the end of the twentieth century, the rich were richer, the poor, poorer. And people everywhere now had a lot less lint, thanks to the lint rollers made in my hometown. It was truly the dawn of a new era

I would like to apologize for referring to George W. Bush as a "deserter." What I meant to say is that George W. Bush is a deserter, an election thief, a drunk driver, a WMD liar, and a functional illiterate. And he poops in his pants.

★ all quotes by Michael Moore in *The Awful Truth*

Jason's Minibar: Truth Serum

When you're ready to unbutton your lip, have a little truth serum and sing like a canary with your fellow expats, because truth is beauty and beauty is truth, and both taste great on the rocks.

Here's what you'll need:
2¼ ounces orange or citrus vodka
¼ ounce Rose's lime juice
Ice
Lemon slice

Here's how you do it:
Put vodka and lime juice in a shaker with lots of ice and shake well. Serve on the rocks, in a cute highball glass, garnished with a thin lemon slice.

▪ *Survivor (2000–)*

This mother of all extreme reality shows deposits sixteen average Americans on an uncharted desert isle, removes or at least hides most of the essentials of comfortable life, including reliable plumbing and drinking water, and waits for *The Lord of the Flies* to start happening. The show's creators even help things along by dividing contestants into two rival tribes, and setting them in competition with each other to become the last man or woman standing and win a million bucks. And while part of this show's appeal is the gross factor when contestants have to do stuff like eat rats, what's most therapeutic about all of the *Survivors* is that people don't turn into savages. Instead, they turn into CEOs making mergers, combining resources, and forming alliances, sometimes with members of the opposing tribe, in order to achieve a common goal. Every *Survivor* has a happy ending, with the man or woman who can remain the calmest under pressure winning the million bucks, and reassuring us all that even if we wind up in the most unforgiving network-contrived reality hell of all time, we can and will survive.

FOOD FOR THOUGHT

Poor as we get in the ghetto, we don't ever eat the rats. Ever.
★ Ramona

You boil it long enough, you can eat anything.
★ Gretchen

When cooking rats, I would imagine that sauce is of the utmost importance.
★ Greg

★ all quotes from *Survivor (2000)*

■ *Curb Your Enthusiasm (2000–)*
Stars: Larry David, Cheryl Hines, Jeff Garlin, Susie Essman

If you're beginning to wonder if everybody else is a member of a private club that hasn't invited you to join, spend a few hours with ultimate outsider Larry David and comfort yourself that as long as he is in the world, there will always be a bigger boor in the room to make you look good.

Larry David of *Seinfeld* fame stars as Larry David, king geek in a kingdom of cool, who spends his life in the throes of a perpetual anxiety attack, because he doesn't play well with others. Larry is a man who has it all: fame, a job he loves, a power agent, a great wife, a beautiful home in the Hollywood Hills, and a fast car. And yet he careens through one socially awkward situation after the next, and always winds up on the short end of the stick, because he just can't seem to relax and go with the flow.

This show, which much like life is a curious hybrid of fact and fiction, reminds us that the best antidote for social anxiety is to remember that even celebrities are insecure people just like the rest of us, so there's really nothing to be afraid of. Although it's probably a good idea to try and avoid staring at your wife's best friend's breasts, alienating your agent's mother, or insulting the president of your network if you want to be popular at your next party. And whatever you do, don't piss off the Starbucks dude. So when you're wrapped tight, unwind with *Curb Your Enthusiasm* and learn from the worst how to be at your best, just by following the golden rule of doing unto others as you would have them do unto you, and yes, that even includes your mother-in-law.

LARRY'S LOWDOWNS

I'll have a vanilla...one of those vanilla bullshit things. You know, whatever you want, some vanilla bullshit latte cappa thing. Whatever you got.

Here's a question for Who Wants to Be a Millionaire?: *what kind of an idiot is running ABC?*

Hear the birds? Sometimes I like to pretend that I'm deaf and I try to imagine what it's like not to be able to hear them. It's not that bad.

Well, I...I thought this was over at death. I didn't know we went into eternity together. Isn't that what it said in...'til death do us part...I guess I had a different plan for eternity. I thought... I thought I'd be single again.

★ all quotes from Larry David as Larry David in *Curb Your Enthusiasm*

WAR, WHAT IS IT GOOD FOR?

If you're dug deep into the trenches and trying to hold on to your nerve just until the reinforcements arrive, come up for air with one of these legendary shows about war buddies who face down the terror of war with the power of compassion, laughter, friendship, and good TV, and remind yourself that true heroes are people just like you, who feel fear, but do the right thing anyway.

Hogan's Heroes (1965–1971)
Stars: Bob Crane, Werner Klemperer, John Banner, Robert Clary, Richard Dawson, Larry Hovis

This zany sixties-style series, which used a German POW camp as the basis for a sitcom, paved the way for the grittier war shows like *M*A*S*H* to come. While Stalag 13 bore absolutely no resemblance to reality, it did demonstrate that under the right circumstances, really horrific situations like a prisoner-of-war camp can be kinda funny, although in this case, the only humor was always at the expense of the enemy.

Colonel Hogan (Bob Crane), the ideal handsome and mischievous good old American bad boy in uniform, and his allied compatriots, who include the French Louis LeBeau (Robert Clary), who knows a lot about cooking, and the British Newkirk (Richard Dawson), who knows a lot about women, spend every episode making mayhem out of Commandant Klink's (Werner Klemperer) best-laid plans. They remind us all that the best antidote to sheer terror is slapstick comedy, bumbling captors, and an underground tunnel that has a fully stocked wine cellar and a two-way transmitter that even broadcasts Radio Free Europe.

KLINK'S KLUNKERS

You can never be nice to a German.
You will not fall in love with anybody until this war is over. That's an order!
Disgraceful. Can't hold their liquor. Can't finish wars they start.

Colonel Klink: Schultz, into the cooler they go. Throw away the key.
Carter: Don't we get a trial or anything?
Colonel Klink: This is Germany. Although I do appreciate
your sense of humor.

Schultz! Close the gates! The war is back on!
★ all quotes from Werner Klemperer as Colonel Klink in *Hogan's Heroes*

LIVE TO TAPE

Robert Clary, who played LeBeau, was a Holocaust survivor. Werner Klemperer, Howard Caine, Leon Askin, and John Banner, who play the Nazis at Stalag 13, were all Jewish.

M*A*S*H (1972–1983)
Stars: Alan Alda, Wayne Rogers, McLean Stevenson,
Loretta Swit, Larry Linville, Gary Burghoff, Mike
Farrell, Harry Morgan, Jamie Farr

The doctors at the 4077th Mobile Army Surgical Hospital (MASH) are on the front lines of the Korean War, attempting to heal the brutality of war with liberal doses of laughter, compassion, camaraderie, free love, and bathtub gin…although not necessarily in that order. The gang includes the anal-retentive and distinctly Republican Major Frank Burns (Larry Linville); the indefatigable Texas tart, Major Margaret "Hot Lips" Houlihan (Loretta Swit), who gives new meaning to the title head nurse; and Corporal Klinger (Jamie Farr), a Greek grunt who serves his country in drag and still can't get dishonorably discharged. And at the head of this encampment of military angels with dirty faces are chief surgeons Hawkeye Pierce (Alan Alda) and Trapper John (Wayne Rogers), who daily go toe-to-toe with war's unending stream of wounded innocents, blind authority, and senseless suffering, and emerge victorious, because they hold on to their humanity, their humility, their sense of humor, their syndication deal, and their three-martini lunches. So if you're feeling like you just can't face another moment on the front lines, let Hawkeye and his merry cohorts remind you that you are stronger than you think you are.

HAWKEYE'S HOMILIES

I will not carry a gun, Frank. When I got thrown into this war I had a clear understanding with the Pentagon: no guns. I'll carry your books, I'll carry a torch, I'll carry a tune, I'll carry on, carry over, carry forward, Cary Grant, cash and carry, carry me back to old Virginia, I'll even "hari-kari" if you show me how, but I will not carry a gun.

No wonder they execute people at dawn. Who wants to live at 6 a.m.?

Did anyone ever tell you, you have the voice of a songbird slowly drowning in tar?

War isn't hell. War is war, and hell is hell. And of the two, war is a lot worse.

★ all quotes from Alan Alda as Hawkeye Pierce in M*A*S*H

TV TIDBITS

The famous *M*A*S*H* theme song was actually a musical contemplation of suicide called "Hail to the Chief, Sayonara." The chorus, which was sung in the movie but omitted in the TV series, is:

Suicide is painless, it brings on many changes
And I can take or leave it as I please.

▪ *In Living Color (1990–1994)*
  Stars: Keenen Ivory Wayans, Jim Carrey, Kelly Coffield, Kim Coles,
  Tommy Davidson, David Alan Grier, T'Keyah Crystal Keymáh,
  Damon Wayans, Kim Wayans, Shawn Wayans, Jamie Foxx,
  Steve Park, Marlon Wayans

Designed as an urban, ethnic answer to the superwhite satire of *Saturday Night Live*, Keenen Ivory Wayans's *In Living Color* reassured all of us in the post-traumatic nineties global village that the mean streets of urban America weren't really so mean after all, once you spent a little time getting to know the hood.

Like the Fly Girl dancers who bumped us in and out of commercial breaks, *In Living Color* is a comedy show with its gloves on and its dukes raised, but its message is ultimately a gentle and a forgiving one, helping ease suburban terrors about the inner city, and letting us all in on the brutality and the mercy of the streets. This was a short-lived series but brought us many long-lasting cultural treasures, like Jim Carrey as the incendiary fire inspector Bill, David Alan Grier as the homoerotically fixated film critic Antoine Merriwether, Damon Wayans as the surly Homey D. Clown, who "don't play that," and Jamie Foxx, who always seemed to be in a dress in the early nineties. Oh, yeah, and there's those Fly Girls, whose hip-hopping ranks included J-Lo in the last season.

In Living Color is TV living out loud, and is a great show to watch when you're experiencing free-floating anxiety about the unknown. The Wayanses and company remind us that the great unknowns that we fear most in life very often turn out to be funny. Even Louis Farrakhan.

Bev's TV Tray: Homeland Security Salad

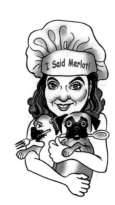

If you're feeling particularly vulnerable to threats from abroad, regain your sense of security with this salad, which proves to you and the world that you know how to take care of number one, because the best defense is to maintain a healthy homeland.

Here's what you'll need:
¼ cup olive oil
1 fennel bulb, white part sliced
6 to 8 shiitake mushrooms
1 red bell pepper
1 yellow bell pepper
2 cloves garlic
¼ cup raspberry or nasturtium vinegar
Dash soy sauce
1 teaspoon Dijon mustard
1 orange
1 lime
1 teaspoon fresh grated ginger
⅛ teaspoon crushed red pepper
Dash sesame oil
Salt and pepper
½ pound mesclun
2 small cans mandarin oranges in their own juice
½ pound fresh mozzarella, cubed

Here's how you do it:

Sauté the fennel and shiitake mushrooms in 1 teaspoon of the olive oil and a little water until they are just slightly softened and set aside. Next, roast peppers at 400 degrees until they pop. Submerge in ice-cold water, then seed and skin them, cut into strips, and drizzle with a little olive oil and 1 clove of minced garlic.

To make the dressing, smash remaining garlic clove into the remaining olive oil in a large bowl. Whisk in the vinegar, soy sauce, mustard, and the juice of 1 orange and 1 lime. Add the ginger, crushed red pepper, sesame oil, and salt and pepper. In a large bowl combine the mesclun, fennel, mushrooms, red and yellow peppers, and mandarin oranges, add cubed mozzarella, and toss with the dressing.

TV JUSTICE

When you're feeling backed into a corner, or lost in a new-millennium frontier where you're making up the rules as you go along, tune in for a little TV justice and reassure yourself that in TV-land at least, the tough questions get asked and answered, the good guys always win, and no villain ever escapes the long arm of the law.

■ *Law & Order* (1990–)
   Stars: Dennis Farina, Jerry Orbach, Sam Waterston, Paul Sorvino, George Dzundza, Jesse L. Martin, Benjamin Bratt, Chris Noth, Michael Moriarty, Elisabeth Rohm, Angie Harmon, Carey Lowell, Jill Hennessy

In *Law & Order* land, sometimes the good guys win and sometimes they don't, but the ultimate victory is always achieved as long as criminals and victims, law and justice, each get their day in court. Taken from actual headlines, each episode begins with a crime investigation that always leads to an arrest, but also always leads to a trial where the system must balance our thirst for moral vengeance with a respect for civil rights and the letter of the law. As these two arms of the criminal justice system battle it out, a portrait emerges of a system that is deeply flawed but essentially sound, and where Lady Liberty manages to keep her eyes wide open in the city that never sleeps. *Law & Order* is a particularly reassuring dose of antianxiety TV medicine because the show takes on troubling current events, and in many cases rescripts reality, so that justice, in TV-land at least, is served up in short order.

LEGAL BRIEFS

Terrific. Now to win a larceny trial all we have to do is prove how the universe ends.
★   Steven Hill as Adam Schiff in *Law & Order*

Reality? The reality is that no one is willing to draw a line in the sand. Nobody is willing to say that the law is the law. And if you break it, you will be prosecuted: win, lose, or draw.
★   Michael Moriarty as Ben Stone in *Law & Order*

Never get Freudian on a man holding a pickle.
★   Sam Waterston as Jack McCoy in *Law & Order*

■ *Judge Judy (1995–)*
Starring: Judge Judy Sheindlin

If you're feeling rattled by the double talk of life, and you're afraid you're going to hit bottom before you can figure out which end is up, spend a few hours with the "judginator," who can always tell the difference between weewee and rainwater, and restore your faith in truth, justice, and the American way.

Judge Judy Sheindlin, a former family court judge in New York City, settles small-claims cases with her signature brand of common sense, a mother's intuition, and a finely honed inner scalpel that always cuts right to the heart of the matter. No matter how petty or heinous the claim, Judy is there to make sure that wrongs are righted, lies are exposed, victims are vindicated, and to reassure us all that there is still some accountability left in a world full of lame excuses.

JUDY'S JUSTICE

Beauty fades. Dumb is forever.

Is the word stupid *written across my forehead?*

I'm speaking. When my mouth moves, yours stops.

Don't spit on my cupcake and tell me it's frosting.
★   all courtroom quotes from *Judge Judy*

■ *Starsky and Hutch (1975–1979)*
Stars: Paul Michael Glaser, David Soul, Antonio Fargas

David Starsky (Paul Michael Glaser) and Ken "Hutch" Hutchinson (David Soul) are two badge-carrying, polyester-wearing badasses, fighting crime, injustice, and the wet look with the help of their monolithic sidekick Huggy Bear (Antonio Fargas), their red Gran Torino, what must be an incredibly powerful blow dryer, and 150-watt smiles on the seventies frontier. And while Starsky and Hutch's methods of law enforcement are definitely a little unorthodox (in one episode Hutch even gets hooked on heroin) and occasionally tread just this side of Ruby Ridge, we know that deep down they are just good buddies trying to do their job, and counting on the strength of their bond to pull them through one of the most morally conflicted cop shows in TV justice history. So if you're feeling unequal to facing the injustice in your world all alone, let Starsky and Hutch remind you that we all need somebody we can lean on, and then call for backup.

■ Oz (1997–2003)

Stars: Kirk Acevedo, Ernie Hudson, Terry Kinney, Rita Moreno,
B. D. Wong, Christopher Maloney, Harold Perrineau, Dean Winters

Jailhouse justice prevails in this brutal and vaguely homoerotic slice-of-life series about life inside the Oswald Maximum Security Penitentiary (hence *Oz*), where justice has already been done and the only morality that remains is survival of the fittest. And while *Oz* is an often harrowing experience to watch, it's a strangely comforting reminder that, as we learn from the prisoners of *Oz*, the toughest bars to break through are the ones inside your skin, and that freedom is just another word for nothing left to fear.

Yeah, I learned the alphabet the hard way. DEA. HIV. IOU.
★ Dean Winters as Ryan O'Reilly in Oz

Remember when your high school history teacher said that the course of human events changes 'cause of the deeds of great men? Well, the bitch was lying. Fuck Caesar, fuck Lincoln, fuck Mahatma Gandhi. The world keeps moving cause of you and me, the anonymous. Revolutions get going 'cause there ain't enough bread. Wars happen over a game of checkers.
★ Harold Perrineau as Augustus Hill in Oz

The Vikings, their brutality aside, had their moments of brilliance. At one point, they were such great shipbuilders that Leif Ericsson and his crew sailed all the way to America. Some people say that he probably went as far down south as the New York harbor. Here's where the brilliance comes in—they took a look and went back.
★ Harold Perrineau as Augustus Hill in Oz

■ *CHiPS* (1977–1983)
   Stars: Erik Estrada, Larry Wilcox

CHiPS followed two adorable motorcycle cops on their daily mission to keep the highways and byways of Los Angeles safe from scum. Officer Frank "Ponch" Poncherello (Erik Estrada) and his more conservative unethnic partner, Officer Jon Baker (Larry Wilcox), whose smile didn't have quite the wattage of Ponch's but who really knew how to fill out a utility belt, came to the rescue of stranded motorists, chased down thieves and thugs, and always managed to win the heart of a damsel in distress—all without ever going in for an oil change or denting a fender. So if you're stuck in idle on the highway of life for fear of the fast lane, let *CHiPS* reassure you that as long as you follow the rules of the road, you'll get to your destination safely.

■ *The Avengers* (1961–1969)
   Stars: Patrick Macnee, Diana Rigg

This cult classic, which seemed to be a British TV James Bond, features John Steed (Patrick Macnee), an agent in Her Majesty's Secret Service, and his partner, Emma Peel (Diana Rigg), who wards off threats to the kingdom without breaking a nail. Steed is an impeccable Englishman, one of the landed gentry in a London Fog and bowler, who can stand calmly in the midst of a full-force gale and never once break wind. His foil is in a Burberry interpretation of a catsuit in black leather, who looks like she has really sharp claws, and can execute a pretty mean flying-tiger-claw kick at the drop of a hat, which can be somewhat unsettling at times to her partner, let alone enemies of the realm. And while this series is definitely short on plot, it's very long on camp appeal and the comforting notion that it really is possible to keep order in the realm without ever once having to break the rules of proper etiquette. John Steed and Emma Peel delivered gentleman's justice.

EMMA'S ESSENTIALS

Always keep your bowler on in time of stress, and watch out for diabolical masterminds.

★ Diana Rigg as Emma Peel in *The Avengers*

■ *Get Smart (1965–1970)*
Stars: Don Adams, Barbara Feldon, Edward Platt

Don Adams stars as Agent Maxwell Smart, America's answer to James Bond and John Steed, who fought comic-book heroes with the help of his sidekick, Agent 99 (Barbara Feldon), a patriarchal boss named Chief (Edward Platt), a convertible Aston Martin, and TV's very first shoe phone. As a secret agent for CONTROL, Max allegorically fought against the forces of KAOS and won, despite the fact that he probably had one of the lowest IQs in TV history, second only to Inspector Jacques Clouseau. Maxwell Smart, who loves danger and knows no fear, really is a symbol of control in a chaotic world, because if Maxwell Smart can get his man, keep his boss and his woman happy, and keep the world free for democracy, then so can you.

MAX'S MOXIE

I may never get to play with the Philharmonic, but on the other hand, is Leonard Bernstein licensed to kill?

What are you talking about, 99? We have to shoot and kill and destroy. We represent everything that's wholesome and good in the world.

★ all quotes from Don Adams as Maxwell Smart in *Get Smart*

▪ *Martha Stewart Living (1991–2004)*

Despite the controversy swirling all around her, Martha, the goddess of good things, manages to keep her eyes focused on the tasks at hand, and while teaching us how to craft and cook, manages to teach us all a little something too: about how to beat anxiety using only a glue gun, a little glitter, and a whole lot of chutzpah.

Despite Martha's sometimes Joan Crawford–esque presence in her signature kitchen, and the impatience she displays with her guests, there is an inner calm about Martha. And as she pinks the edge of a lavender sachet, or arranges a salmon fillet on a bed of grape twigs, she is not just cooking and crafting but representing her brand of kitchen Zen, which counsels that when we're chopping a cabbage we should just chop the cabbage, and just forget about the SEC, no matter what the NBC anchor on our left shoulder is saying to distract us. So the next time the wolf is at your front door, keep him at bay with some of Martha's comfort-food TV, and then open your door, invite the wolf in for dinner, and make friends with your fear.

CHAPTER 9

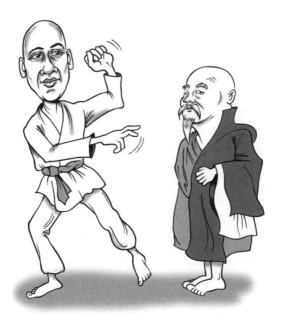

TV for the Soul

IF YOU'RE BEGINNING TO wonder if this is all there is, and you're hungry for deeper meaning, rise above with a little TV for the Soul and kick-start your joie de vivre. These TV shows remind us that true beauty seldom lies right on the surface, and encourage us to look more deeply and sensitively at our own world, by showing us worlds we've never seen before.

▪ *Medium* (2005–)
  Stars: *Patricia Arquette, Miguel Sandoval, Sofia Vassilieva, Jake Weber,*
    Craig Gellis, Maria Lark

Psychic soccer mom Alison Dubois (Patricia Arquette, straight from *Stigmata*) brings a whole new meaning to the concept of work/life balance as she struggles to fulfill her roles as a wife and mom, while simultaneously solving crimes through her connection with the spirit world. Yes, it's true; Alison sees dead people, and even sometimes hears the thoughts of the people around her, which can be a mixed bag in a marriage. Fortunately, she's also got a bad memory, which is probably a blessing. Driven by impulses from the hereafter and working-mom's guilt in the here and now, Alison uses her sixth sense to solve crimes and still makes it home to have dinner on the table for her daughter—who fortunately or unfortunately shares her mom's gift of second sight. Based on the real-life story of research medium Alison Dubois, *Medium* reminds all of us who are wondering if this is all there is, that there is definitely more to life than meets the eye, even lying just beneath the surface in the most superficial suburban plane.

▪ *Kung Fu* (1972–1975)
  Stars: *David Carradine, Keye Luke, Barry Sullivan, Richard Loo,*
    Phillip Ahn

If you're having difficulty hearing yourself think, spend a few hours with Kwai Chang Caine (David Carradine), the East-meets-West mystic who reminds us to stop and hear the grasshoppers. Long before crouching tigers and hidden dragons, Kwai Chang Caine, the inscrutable Shaolin priest from the East with the power of the tiger, the wings of a dragon, and Clint Eastwood's five-mile squint, lifted us up out of the hubbub of noisy modern life and carried us away to a TV nirvana, where love overpowers loud.

Raised in a Shaolin monastery by the blind Master Po (Keye Luke), young Caine, nicknamed "Grasshopper," absorbs the wisdom of the ages by doing really cool things like walking across hot coals and sparring with sticks. When fate forces him to avenge his master's murder, his path leads him from the well-trodden paths of Tibet to blaze new trails in the wild wild West. In the American frontier, Caine walks softly carrying a big stick, and confronts crudeness with kindness, violence with forgiveness, and hatred with love, in an effort to atone for his own sins, most notable of which was stealing the part from a real Asian guy.

But for all of us urban cowboys and girls in the seventies and now, who have taken a few kicks to the rear and are ready to get out of the rodeo, *Kung Fu* is welcome relief from the blazing saddles of the Western world, and transports us, for a few hours anyway, into a peaceful coexistence where the biggest challenge is trying to snatch a pebble from an old man's hand.

CAINE'S CORNERSTONES

The courageous fighter shuns violence. The skillful soldier avoids anger. A mighty warrior does not fight for petty conquests.

A battle avoided cannot be lost.

One gathers friends with many skills in fifteen years of wandering.

In kung fu, battle does not force you apart. It brings you together.
★ all quotes from David Carradine as Kwai Chang Caine in *Kung Fu*

LIVE TO TAPE

Kung Fu was originally created as a vehicle for Bruce Lee, but producers insisted that an Asian could not command a large enough audience, and David Carradine was cast in the role.

▪ *A Year in Provence* (1993)
   Stars: John Thaw, Lindsay Duncan

If you're longing to escape to a more fundamental and soulful place, where all of life can be summed up in a spoonful of peasant soup, spend a few hours with Peter (John Thaw) and Annie Mayle (Lindsay Duncan), who left their modern urban life behind to spend a year in the French countryside. As they learn to cook and enjoy the regional foods, and breathe in the soulful atmosphere of Provence, they, and we along with them, begin to understand why the French make such great spirits. This miniseries is like a TV picnic in the open air, with a stinky cheese and a good bottle of red wine.

GUYS THAT FLY

Saturday Night Live: The Best of Chris Farley (1998)
Chris Farley, with his jolly physique and clumsy comedy, quickly became our favorite *Saturday Night Live* player because he was completely unashamed of his own dorkdom.

Whether he was living in a van down by the river, dancing in tights, or bugging celebrities in an elevator, Chris could always crack us up because he not only embraced his inner geek, he got all four-hundred-plus pounds of him to fly.

Saturday Night Live: The Best of Will Ferrell (2002)
It's true, few comedians can pull off being Janet Reno, President Bush, James Lipton, *and* Craig the obsessive flying cheerleader without breaking a funny bone or two. But the thing we love best about *The Best of Will Ferrell* is that this is a man with a gut like the rest of us, and some weird scar that we still haven't gotten to the bottom of, who is completely unafraid to get undressed on national television. Will Ferrell's naked lunch fuels all of our hopes for a better tomorrow, when even those of us without six-pack abs can go vaulting over our body-image hurdles and defy gravity.

▪ *Antiques Roadshow (1997)*

A team of antiques experts and appraisers tours the country and lets all of the collectors who live in the area bring in the weird junk that they've collected through the years, and the experts tell them if they've got trash or treasure. Some people really do wind up with treasure, like a collection of presidential autographs dating from George Washington, a nineteenth-century Navajo blanket appraised at $350,000, and a mahogany coffee table that was in some lady's basement in New Jersey that she later sold at Sotheby's for half a million bucks. But aside from the great education we get about the soulful hobby of antiquing, it also reminds us to take a closer look at the tiny details that surround us unnoticed every day, because they could be priceless treasures.

OUT-OF-THE-WORLD TV

Because sometimes in order to appreciate your world, you have to leave it behind and expand your horizons.

Star Trek (*1966–1969*)
Stars: William Shatner, Leonard Nimoy, DeForest Kelley, George Takei, Nichelle Nichols, James Doohan, Walter Koenig

If you're in the mood to boldly go where no man—or woman—has gone before, but you've lost your moral compass, report to the bridge of the USS *Enterprise*, and let Captain Kirk (William Shatner) and his crew remind you of the prime directive and put you back on course. This series, which is a landmark cult classic that has inspired millions around the globe to dress up in funny double-knit T-shirts and put on fake pointy ears, is like an episodic morality lesson about the dangers of manifest destiny, and cautions us all that while it's fine to visit a brave new world, we have to respect the integrity of the cultures we encounter, or risk being hurled into a time warp with an inactivated phaser bank, facing with no security shield a butt load of angry Klingons.

In the course of just four seasons, *Star Trek* managed to tackle most of the ponderous moral and ethical conflicts of the ages. Without the benefit of digitalization or any real special effects, *Star Trek* manages to hold our attention as Captain Kirk and his first mate, Spock (Leonard Nimoy), play out their mini-epic Greek tragedies and resolve the conflicts of the ages in just under sixty minutes, not including commercial interruptions. *Star Trek* wrestled with most of the big questions facing us on our spiritual path and boiled them down to one golden rule. Guided by the prime directive, the crew of the USS *Enterprise* finds a way to balance reason against passion, and choose tolerance over prejudice, peace over war, patience over provocation. And while these cosmic morality plays are set on faraway and exotic worlds, populated by aliens, and costumed with some of the most imaginative ensembles to ever visit the planet polyester, the issues that confront us feel just like home.

So if you're feeling like a stalled starship in an increasingly volatile quadrant, and you're wondering how you can summon your inner warp drive and navigate your way to a better world, let Scotty beam you back up to the *Enterprise*, a sixties vision of multinational utopia where the only mandate is peace.

WORDS TO LIVE BY

Those of you who have served for long on this vessel have encountered alien life-forms. You know the greatest danger facing us is ourselves and irrational fear of the unknown. But there's no such thing as "the unknown," only things temporarily hidden, temporarily not understood.
★ William Shatner as Captain Kirk in *Star Trek*

We need no urging to hate humans, but for the present, only a fool fights in a burning house.
★ Michael Ansara as Kang in *Star Trek*

Spock, I've found that evil usually triumphs...unless good is very, very careful.
★ DeForest Kelley as Dr. McCoy in *Star Trek*

Angel (*1999–2004*)

Stars: David Boreanaz, Charisma Carpenter, Glenn Quinn

What better place to find an angel than in the city of angels, where gods and monsters roam the midnight alleyways unfettered and free to work their will on the unwitting citizens of Tinsel Town. Fortunately, Angel (David Boreanaz), who isn't really an angel at all but a vampire in recovery (not to mention Buffy's ex-boyfriend), has vowed to regain his humanity by fighting evil wherever it lurks, and saving the souls of lost and helpless Angelenos. So he sets up a detective agency with his sidekick, Cordelia (Charisma Carpenter), a frustrated actress with a great pair of gams who wants to be loved for her mind, and his half-human partner, Doyle (Glenn Quinn). Together these otherworldly crusaders, who seem to have stepped straight out of a neonoir novel, take on the forces of evil and rescue the helpless from the monsters that threaten to devour them.

Dark Shadows (*1966–1971*)

Stars: Jonathan Frid, Grayson Hall, David Selby

If your backyard is looking a lot like an unweeded garden that's gone to seed, and you're ready to shuffle off your mortal coil for a few hours, let the reluctant immortals of Collinswood Manor remind you that it's a wonderful life, and that no one who still has a pulse is poor.

Conflicted vampire Barnabas Collins (Jonathan Frid), who is clearly a spiritual father of Anne Rice's tormented Louis, the vampire with the soul of a human (although Barnabas does not, like Louis, have the face of Brad Pitt), stalks the dark shadows of his haunted family home in search of the love and humanity he lost two centuries ago. Desperate for even a few moments of mortality, he manipulates the world around him with characteristic vampire charm. And in doing so, Barnabas somehow managed to steal the hearts of prepubescent American girls in the sixties, who for some reason got a real charge out of an aging and myopic British actor in a cape and way too much black eyeliner, with big pointy teeth and a complete inability to remember his lines.

Meanwhile, Quentin (David Selby), the tortured Heathcliffian bad boy who is always in a state about something, poisons the world around him with his desperate need for a reliable love that can rescue him from himself. Needless to say, he also made the cover of *Teen Beat*. And then there's Dr. Julia (Grayson Hall), the perpetually overlooked Collins daughter, who becomes a blood disorder specialist in order to heal the psychic wounds of her dysfunctional family of origin and get the validation she craves from her mother and Barnabas. If this sounds something like the last supernatural thriller that took place in your family room, you're right. Together with a whole host of gothic ghouls and goblins, the Collinses shine a different light on the petty soap operas of daily life and show us that even the scariest monsters are just poor and misunderstood souls who can't quite remember their dialogue, all desperately looking for love in all the wrong places, while trying to keep one eye on the teleprompter.

COLLINSWOOD CONUNDRUMS

Time is a rushing, howling wind that rages past me, withering me in a single, relentless blast, and then continues on. I've been sitting here passively, submissive to its rage, watching its work. Listen! Time, howling, withering!

★ Jonathan Frid as Barnabas Collins in *Dark Shadows*

Men change. And seldom for the better.

★ Joan Bennett as Elizabeth Collins in *Dark Shadows*

Angelique, we cannot love at will, any more than we can prevent our love.

★ Jonathan Frid as Barnabas Collins in *Dark Shadows*

I don't want a sedative! I want Jeb!

★ Nancy Barrett as Carolyn Collins in *Dark Shadows*

If only we could find a way of telling the truth without anyone knowing what actually happened.

★ David Selby as Quentin Collins in *Dark Shadows*

■ *All Creatures Great and Small (1978–1990)*
   Stars: Christopher Timothy, Robert Hardy, Peter Davison,
      Carol Drinkwater, Lynda Bellingham

Based on the best-selling book series by James Herriot, this series follows the ups and downs of a veterinarian in Yorkshire, England, in the 1940s. This real-life Dr. Dolittle leaves city life behind for the slow and soulful pace of a small farming community, whose residents are a little suspicious about their new vet. Thankfully, Dr. Herriot (Christopher Timothy) is championed by the old vet in town, Siegfried Garnon (Robert Hardy), who schools the young man in the ways of animals and people, and reminds us that all good things come to those who wait, and that life and death are in the details.

DISASTERTHERAPY

Airline *(2004)*

Set in Los Angeles International Airport and Chicago's Midway Airport, this reality show follows the trials and tribulations of Southwest Airlines customer service personnel as they attempt to solve just about every human dilemma, petty and profound, and still manage to get their planes to the runway on time. Facing issues ranging from body odor to belligerence to too many tugs on the bottle, these ministering angels of customer comfort and passenger safety must find quick and wrinkle-free solutions to pressing problems, negotiate compromises among warring factions, and pull the troublemakers off their flights without inciting a riot. Watching this show reminds us that you can't expect to take off until you get your own clay feet off the ground.

▪ *Psychic Detectives (1992)*

If you're feeling like your unanswered questions have been pushed to the back of the filing cabinet of life, let these psychic detectives help you turn up a new lead by learning to trust your instincts.

Real-life cases that baffle traditional investigators are turned over to psychics, who can sense the energy of murder and trauma, and follow the astral trail of trauma, leading detectives to the location of the bodies they have been searching for. While it is true that all of these psychics are slightly rotund women who wear a lot of purple, their visions are so accurate that they soften even the hardest hometown-cop critics, who don't believe in anything that they can't slap ketchup on and eat for lunch. In addition to being some gripping rubberneck TV, it's reassuring to realize that no matter what you're trying to solve, when you've reached a dead end, you can always reach outside of the box and find a new direction.

Jason's Minibar

Joy Juice
Spread a little love with this delicious nonalcoholic punch, and let all the sunshine in.

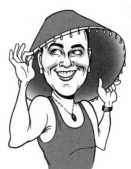

Here's what you'll need:
6 ounces orange juice concentrate
6 ounces lemonade concentrate
1 quart chilled apple juice
2 quarts chilled ginger ale
1 pint lemon sherbet
Ice

Here's how you do it:
Mix the orange juice, lemonade, and apple juice into a punch bowl. Stir the ginger ale into the bowl. Spoon in sherbet and then gather the crew and ring dem bells.

ANGELS AND DEMONS

In TV-land, as in life, it can sometimes be hard to tell the difference between the powers of good and the forces of darkness. Angels don't always wear halos, and devils don't always have horns. In fact, sometimes, it's vice versa. So if you're in the grip of something that's larger than you, or you're having trouble telling friend from foe, let these demons with hearts of gold and angels with dirty faces reassure you that good will always triumph over evil, as long as you trust yourself.

Charlie's Angels *(1976–1981)*
Stars: Farrah Fawcett, Kate Jackson, Jaclyn Smith, David Doyle,
    John Forsythe

If you're feeling weighed down by the petty misdemeanors of everyday life, spend a few hours with Sabrina (Kate Jackson), Jill (Farrah Fawcett), and Kelly (Jaclyn Smith), three law-enforcing angels on earth who will carry you away to a braless, lip gloss heaven, where every wrong is righted with a crisp karate kick and a quick phone call to God, followed by a full-screen derriere shot.

In this seventies-style babe-alicious vision of a TV hereafter, God is Charlie Townsend (John Forsythe), an offscreen rich guy with a dynastic voice that's a cross between John Carrington in *Dynasty* and Donald Trump, and a speakerphone with great range. His right-hand man is John Bosley (David Doyle), a chubby yes-man in a bad suit, and his angels are three cover girls in skimpy synthetics who really know how to work their wings. Yet despite the alarming highlights, and the obvious lack of supportive underwires, these angels manage to vanquish evil and champion good wherever their platform pumps take them and reassure us that sometimes, if you want to get to heaven, you've got to raise a little hell.

Charmed *(1998–)*
Stars: Shannen Doherty, Holly Marie Combs, Alyssa Milano

When sisters Pru (Shannen Doherty), Piper (Holly Marie Combs), and Phoebe (Alyssa Milano) Halliwell find the Book of Shadows and discover that they are actually witches, all hell breaks loose in their suburban neighborhood until the gals get to know their own strengths. They learn that while each has her own unique specialty—Pru can move objects, Piper freezes time, Phoebe sees the future—their greatest power lies in the magical power of three. Their combined force can slay dragons and vanquish demons, and still manage to get a date to the prom. Those witches remind us that all you need to live a charmed life is to keep moving toward the light.

Bev's TV Tray: A Little Taste of Heaven

Just like TV has tried to show us what heaven and angels might look and feel like, great chefs have tried to imagine what paradise would taste like. Here are a few of my favorite culinary metaphors for the sweet hereafter.

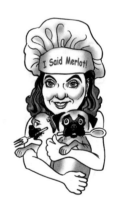

Paradise Pudding

Here's what you'll need:
   $1/4$ cup blanched almonds
   12 marshmallows
   12 candied cherries
   6 macaroons
   1 package lemon Jell-O
   1 cup whipped cream, plus extra for garnish
   $1/4$ cup sugar

Here's how you do it:

Dice almonds, marshmallows, cherries, and macaroons and set aside. Make the lemon Jell-O and set aside to cool in fridge. When the Jell-O is cold but not quite set, fold in whipped cream, nut and fruit mixture, and sugar. Chill until set and serve with a little more whipped cream and a cherry on top.

Divinity

Here's what you'll need:
   $^{1}/_{2}$ cup light corn syrup
   $2^{1}/_{2}$ cups sugar
   $^{1}/_{4}$ teaspoon salt
   $^{1}/_{2}$ cup water
   2 egg whites
   1 teaspoon vanilla
   1 cup chopped walnuts

Here's how you do it:

Combine corn syrup, sugar, salt, and water in a saucepan and cook at low heat until the sugar is dissolved. Leave on the heat without stirring until a small amount of the mixture forms a ball when dropped in cold water. Next, beat the egg whites until they're stiff. Pour about half of the sugar syrup over the egg whites, whisking constantly. Cook the remainder of the sugar syrup until a small amount forms threads in cold water. Then add this slowly to the egg white mixture and whisk until it holds its shape. Add vanilla and fold in walnuts, then spread in a greased pan, and when cool, cut into squares.

Ambrosia

Here's what you'll need:
 3 oranges, peeled and sectioned
 4 to 6 teaspoons sugar
 3 bananas, sliced thinly
 1 cup shredded coconut, unsweetened

Here's how you do it:
Cover the bottom of a glass bowl with the orange sections. Sprinkle some of the sugar over the oranges, then cover with a layer of bananas. Sprinkle some of the coconut over the bananas. Continue layering fruit, sugar, and coconut until you've used all the fruit. Finish with a layer of coconut and refrigerate for an hour before serving.

INDEX

D

H

I

J

N

O

P